W9-BNS-142

Love & Survival

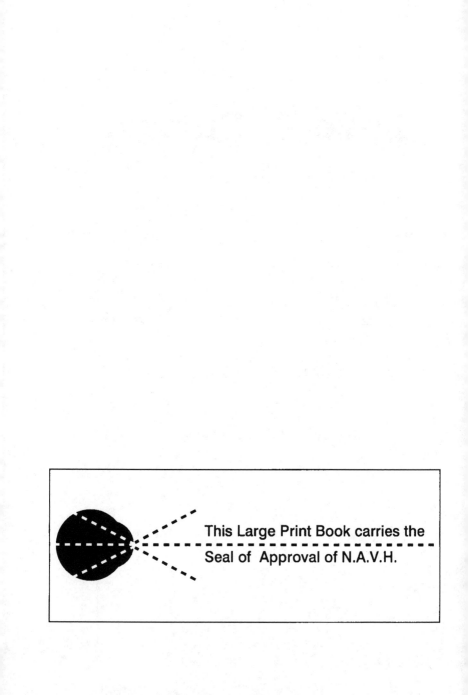

This Large Print Book carries the
Seal of Approval of N.A.V.H.

Love & Survival

The Scientific Basis for the Healing Power of Intimacy

Dean Ornish, M.D.

Thorndike Press • Thorndike, Maine

The quotation by James Pennebaker is reprinted with permission of James Pennebaker, currently a professor at University of Texas at Austin, from his book *Opening Up: The Healing Power of Expressing Emotion.* New York: Guilford Press, 1997.

The interview with Ralph Fiennes is reprinted with permission of *Parade,* copyright © 1997.

The excerpt from the article by L.F. Berkman, "The Role of Social Relations in Health Promotion," published in volume 57, 1995, pp. 245–54 of *Psychosomatic Medicine,* is reprinted with permission of Williams and Wilkins.

The illustration on page 64 is reprinted with permission of Williams and Wilkins. It is taken from page 148 of *Psychosomatic Medicine,* volume 59 (2), published 1997.

Published in 1998 by arrangement with HarperCollins Publishers, Inc.

Thorndike Large Print ® Americana Series.

The tree indicium is a trademark of Thorndike Press.

The text of this Large Print edition is unabridged.
Other aspects of the book may vary from the original edition.

Set in 16 pt. Plantin by Juanita Macdonald.

Printed in the United States on permanent paper.

Library of Congress Cataloging in Publication Data

Ornish, Dean.
    Love & survival : the scientific basis for the healing power of intimacy / Dean Ornish.
       p. cm.
    Originally published: New York : HarperCollins, 1998.
    Includes bibliographical references.
    ISBN 0-7862-1550-X (lg. print : hc : alk. paper)
    1. Love.   2. Intimacy (Psychology)   3. Longevity.
4. Health.   5. Large type books.   I. Title.
[RC685.C6O757   1998]
   613—dc21   98-26645

For Molly

If they can get you to ask the wrong questions, then they don't have to worry about the answers.

— Thomas Pynchon, *Gravity's Rainbow*

Think different.

— Apple Computer

Contents

Contents

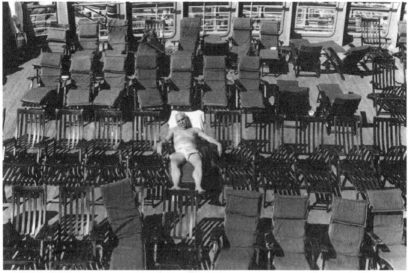

QE2, 1971

1

Love and Survival

Love and survival.

What do they have to do with each other?

This book is based on a simple but powerful idea: Our survival depends on the healing power of love, intimacy, and relationships. Physically. Emotionally. Spiritually. As individuals. As communities. As a country. As a culture. Perhaps even as a species.

Most people tend to think of my work as being primarily about diet. It's gotten to the point where it's hard for me to go out to dinner with people without them apologizing for what they're eating or making comments about my food — even though I make it clear that I'm not the food police.

Many stories have appeared in the media about the research I have directed for the past twenty years that has demonstrated, for the first time, that comprehensive lifestyle changes may begin to reverse even severe coronary heart disease without drugs or surgery. Almost always, these articles focus on my diet: "What do people eat?" "Isn't this diet too strict for most people?" "Are they going to live longer or is it just going to *seem* longer?" And so on.

I have no intention of diminishing the power of diet and exercise or, for that matter, of drugs and surgery. There is more scientific evidence now than ever before demonstrating how simple changes in diet and lifestyle may cause significant improvements in health and well-being. As important as these are, I have found that perhaps the most powerful intervention — and the most meaningful for me and for most of the people with whom I work, including staff and patients — is the healing power of love and intimacy, and the emotional and spiritual transformation that often result from these. While I have written about these themes in my earlier books, the emotional and spiritual aspects of disease tend to get overlooked — so I decided to write an entire book on the subject.

In this book, I describe the increasing scientific evidence from my own research and from the studies of others that cause me to believe that love and intimacy are among the most powerful factors in health and illness, even though these ideas are largely ignored by the medical profession. As I review the extensive scientific literature that supports these ideas, I will describe the limitations of science to document and understand the full range of these implications — not only in our health and illness, but also in what often brings the most joy, value, and meaning to our lives. I give examples from my life and from the lives of friends, colleagues, and patients.

Medicine today tends to focus primarily on the physical and mechanistic: drugs and surgery, genes and germs, microbes and molecules. *I am not aware of any other factor in medicine — not diet, not smoking, not exercise, not stress, not genetics, not drugs, not surgery — that has a greater impact on our quality of life, incidence of illness, and premature death from all causes.*

Cholesterol, for example, is clearly related to the incidence of illness and premature death from heart disease and stroke. Those with the highest blood cholesterol levels may have a risk of heart attack several times greater than those with the lowest levels, and lowering cholesterol levels will reduce the risk of heart disease and stroke. However, cholesterol levels are not related to such diseases as complications during pregnancy and childbirth, the incidence of illness and premature death from infectious diseases, arthritis, ulcers, and so on, whereas loneliness and isolation may significantly increase the risk of all these. Something else is going on.

Smoking, diet, and exercise affect a wide variety of illnesses, but no one has shown that quitting smoking, exercising, or changing diet can double the length of survival in women with metastatic breast cancer, whereas the enhanced love and intimacy provided by weekly group support sessions has been shown to do just that, as I will describe in chapter 2.[1] While genetics plays a role in most illnesses, the number of diseases in which our genes play a primary, causative role is relatively small. Genetic factors — even when combined with cholesterol levels

12

and all of the known risk factors — account for no more than one-half the risk of heart disease.

Love and intimacy are at a root of what makes us sick and what makes us well, what causes sadness and what brings happiness, what makes us suffer and what leads to healing. If a new drug had the same impact, virtually every doctor in the country would be recommending it for their patients. It would be malpractice not to prescribe it — yet, with few exceptions, we doctors do not learn much about the healing power of love, intimacy, and transformation in our medical training. Rather, these ideas are often ignored or even denigrated.

It has become increasingly clear to even the most skeptical physicians why diet is important. Why exercise is important. Why stopping smoking is important. But love and intimacy? Opening your heart? And what *is* emotional and spiritual transformation?

I am a scientist. I believe in the value of science as a powerful means of gaining greater understanding of the world we live in. Science can help us sort out truth from fiction, hype from reality, what works from what doesn't work, for whom, and under what circumstances. Although I respect the ways and power of science, I also understand its limitations as well. What is most meaningful often cannot be measured. What is verifiable may not necessarily be what is most important. As the British scientist Denis Burkitt once wrote, "Not everything that counts can be counted."

We may not yet have the tools to measure what is most meaningful to people, but the value of those experiences is not diminished by our inability to quantify them. We can listen, we can learn, and we can benefit greatly from those who have had these experiences. When we gather together to tell and listen to each other's stories, the sense of community and the recognition of shared experiences can be profoundly healing.

I am fascinated by the increasing interest in alternative medicine yet concerned that many of these remedies have little scientific evidence to support their use. I am continually amazed by the success of books making the most astonishing claims — for example, that bacon and eggs are good for you if you have a particular blood type — by authors who have never conducted or even cited a single scientific research study to support their unfounded claims even when they may be misleading and even harmful.

There is intense interest at all levels in controlling health care costs. Managed-care organizations are trying to control costs by shortening hospital stays, limiting reimbursement, shifting from inpatient to outpatient surgery, and forcing doctors to see more and more patients in less and less time — none of which addresses the more fundamental lifestyle factors that are such powerful determinants of why people get sick and why they often have a hard time changing their lifestyles. Both doctors and patients are increasingly frustrated.

Many physicians complain that it's not a lot of fun to practice medicine these days, and the quality of care is often compromised. According to recent surveys, most doctors would not recommend medicine as a career to their sons or daughters — a telling indictment of our profession. Many physicians are finding that practicing medicine only as a technician, mechanic, or plumber does not feed their souls any more than it leaves patients feeling nourished in the ways that most matter.

Dr. Mimi Guarneri is an interventional cardiologist who directs a reversing-heart-disease program, based on my work, at the Scripps Clinic and Hospital in La Jolla, California. She spends part of her time performing angioplasties and part of her time teaching her patients how to change their lifestyle.

"I recently gave a lecture to a large group of cardiologists," she told me. "At first, I talked with them about radioactive stents, a wire mesh designed to keep angioplastied arteries open by exposing them to high doses of localized radiation. Although it's a new, totally unproven method with the possibility of highly toxic long-term side effects, the cardiologists just *loved* the idea of these radioactive stents. They *couldn't wait* to try them. In the second half of my presentation I talked about our lifestyle program. Even though we have twenty years of randomized controlled trial data supporting your program, the cardiologists got so skeptical and even hostile to the idea that patients could change their lifestyle and that emotions play a role in health and illness that many left the room."

Along the same lines, about two years ago I gave a lecture to more than five thousand cardiologists who make their living performing angioplasty — about why diet and lifestyle may sometimes be a better choice than angioplasty. Not exactly the most receptive audience. I was introduced by the director of the conference, Dr. Martin Leon, an internationally admired interventional cardiologist, who said, "You're probably wondering why I invited Dean Ornish to speak at a conference on aggressive interventional cardiology. Well, because his program *is* aggressive interventional cardiology of a different type."

The irony is this: At a time when there is so much scientific evidence about the importance of spending time talking with people about their lifestyle and psychosocial factors, most doctors have neither the time nor training to do it. If a physician has to see a new patient every eight minutes, he or she doesn't have time to talk about the problems at home with the wife or the husband or the kid on drugs or whatever the stress happens to be at work. There is time only to listen to the heart and lungs, write a prescription, and go on to the next patient.

This frustration, in part, is why interest in alternative medicine is growing so rapidly. According to the *New England Journal of Medicine*, more money is spent out of pocket for alternative medicine than for traditional medicine — even though most insurance companies do not yet cover these costs.[2]

Why?

The desire for connection and caring is so compelling that many people will pay out of their own pocket in order to have these needs met. Doctors who make fun of these "touchy-feely" practices ignore these basic human needs at their own economic risk.

Patients are voting with their feet. As a result, even conservative and prestigious medical schools are beginning to add alternative medicine (also known as "integrative medicine") programs to their curricula. This would not have happened even a few years ago.

At the School of Medicine, University of California, San Francisco (UCSF), for example, I am a cofounder of the new Center for Integrative Medicine. In this program, we are teaching and studying innovative approaches in medicine that integrate the best of traditional and nontraditional approaches to health and healing to medical students, interns, residents, fellows, practicing physicians, nurses, and other health professionals.

Whatever the differences in modalities of alternative medicine provided — acupuncture, yoga, massage, chiropractic, therapeutic touch, for example — what almost all integrative medicine practices have in common is that the practitioners spend time with their patients, they listen to them, and they often touch and help them feel nurtured and nourished.

In 1977, when I was a second-year medical student, I began conducting research to determine if the progression of even severe coronary heart disease may be reversible. At that time, the idea that heart disease was reversible was considered impossible by most doctors. It was hard even to get funding to do the research — "Why should we waste our money funding research that we know can't possibly work?" It was a catch-22: Without the funding, we couldn't do the research to see if it was possible to reverse heart disease; since most funding agencies thought it was impossible, they didn't want to support the research.

Now, this "impossible" idea has become mainstream. *Why* heart disease is reversible, though, has been the subject of much debate.

In a series of randomized controlled trials, my colleagues and I used high-tech, state-of-the-art technology to assess the power of ancient, low-tech, and low-cost interventions. We found that even severe heart disease often can begin healing in only a few weeks, without drugs or surgery. Using tests such as thallium scans, radionuclide ventriculograms, and cardiac PET scans, we measured overall improvement in blood flow to the heart and in the ability of the heart to pump blood; using computer-analyzed quantitative coronary arteriograms, we found that even severely blocked coronary arteries became measurably less blocked.[3–24]

As important as these findings were, most of these research participants and their families said that even more meaningful to them were changes that were more difficult to quantify:

- Rediscovering inner sources of peace, joy, and well-being
- Learning how to communicate in ways that enhanced intimacy with loved ones
- Creating a healthy community of friends and family
- Developing more compassion and empathy for themselves and others
- Experiencing directly the transcendent interconnectedness of life

When I have presented our research findings at scientific meetings, many of the other physicians and scientists told me that they believed the benefits of my program were due solely to diet and exercise. They thought that the stress management techniques and group support had little, if any, benefit. The fact that there are many well-done studies demonstrating the role of emotional stress in heart disease made little difference to them; neither did our finding that adherence to the stress management techniques was as strongly correlated with changes in coronary artery disease as was adherence to the diet.

Even those who believed that cholesterol is important often asked, "Why bother to change your diet and lifestyle when you can just take a pill to lower your cholesterol? Cholesterol-lowering drugs can help reverse heart disease, too."

Medications can be very useful in some cases, but they may not be the best first choice. Why take powerful drugs for the rest of your life to lower cholesterol when you can often achieve similar results with diet and lifestyle at a fraction of the cost — literally billions of dollars per year — and without the known and unknown side effects? The only side effects of changing diet and lifestyle are good ones. Also, the same diet that can help reverse heart disease also may help prevent prostate cancer, breast cancer, colon cancer, lymphoma, osteoporosis, diabetes, hypertension, arthritis, and obesity.

In addition, pills to lower cholesterol do not make you feel better. Comprehensive changes in diet and lifestyle cause most people to feel so much better, so quickly, that it reframes the reason for changing from risk factor modification or living a few months longer or fear of dying to increasing the joy of living.

More important, taking pills to lower cholesterol without addressing the psychological, emotional, and spiritual dimensions of health and healing misses an opportunity to transform one's life in ways that make it more joyful and meaningful.

If you were to look up *stress* in the index of summaries of one of these scientific presentations — at the annual scientific session of the American Heart Association or the American College of Cardiology, for example — you would find *stress echocardiography, exercise stress testing,* and *stress Doppler testing,* but very little about emotional stress or any other psychological factors, and nothing at all on the spiritual dimensions of the heart — even though the heart has been the symbol of love, compassion, emotions, and spirituality for thousands of years. *Love* is not even in the index. You might think that *love* would be in the domain of psychologists, yet a review of the *Annual Review of Psychology* (twenty-three volumes!) found not a single reference to love.[25]

When I searched the National Library of Medicine database from 1966 to 1997, I found 6,059,652 research publications under *human,* 277,175 under *heart,* 2,205 under *love,* but only four articles that mentioned both love and heart disease. Of these four articles, one was on the inventor of a new technology in pediatric cardiology and his "love both of good times and difficult problems" and one was a Japanese article on how heart transplants should be offered "out of love for mankind." Only two of more than nine million articles in the National Library of Medicine Database described the relationship of love to heart disease.

As recently as May 1997, an article in the *Journal of the American Medical Association* reviewed all of the known risk factors for coronary heart disease.[26] While listing esoteric factors such as apolipoprotein E isoforms, cholesteryl ester transfer protein, and lecithin-cholesterol acyl transferase, it did not even mention emotional stress or other psychosocial factors, much less spiritual ones.

I want to make it clear that I am not at all against the use of drugs and surgery; when used appropriately, they may have great value. I prescribe cholesterol-lowering medications and other drugs and refer people for surgery if, for whatever reason, they are not interested in making comprehensive lifestyle changes or if they need help in addition to these changes. We do not know if patients may experience even more improvement by including lipid-lowering drugs plus comprehensive lifestyle changes. Also, in a crisis, drugs and surgery can be lifesaving.

In May 1995, I ran in a seven-and-a-half mile race called the "Bay to Breakers." It's a very San Francisco kind of race. Serious runners compete alongside with people dressed in drag or wearing costumes — or nothing at all. I usually run only about two to three miles at a time, so by the sixth mile I was getting tired and looking for an excuse to slow down. At that moment, I was surprised to see a man lying motionless on the ground — a good excuse.

I helped perform CPR with another doctor and we administered intravenous medications. Some paramedics brought a defibrillator and we were able to shock the man's heart and get it started again, and he was taken to the hospital where he underwent emergency bypass surgery.

I went on to finish the race; at the end, they gave everyone a T-shirt that said, "I survived the Bay to Breakers race," so I stopped by the hospital and gave it to the man as a souvenir. Interestingly, he is a high school English teacher in Seattle, and the surgery was performed by one of his former high school students.

Of course, I didn't feed him vegetables or teach him how to meditate when he was lying in the street; there is a time and a place for drugs and surgery. Even when these are necessary, they are just the beginning. We can then ask, "What can be learned from this experience? How did you get in this position? What can you do to help keep it from happening again?"

After recovering from bypass surgery, this man came and spent a week with my colleagues and me at one of our weeklong retreats to reduce the likelihood of ever needing to undergo another cardiac operation. At the end of the retreat, his wife gave me a beautiful poem that I now keep over my desk:

The Race

A message burns the wires:
    he's had a heart attack.
My world goes black;
    blood plummets to my feet.
Just blocks away,
    the seven-mile human ribbon ripples
lazily as thousands throng
    the streets of San Francisco
walking, jogging, joking, pushing prams,
    He made it
over Heartbreak Hill, past the Panhandle,
    into the Park
then fell. His heart stopped,
    full cardiac arrest, dead,

25

in any other time or place;
    but synchronicity, coincidence,
miracle or fate,
    whatever name we give to forces
that we cannot understand,
    gave him another chance.

If we lived back in ancient Greece
    where gods personify
these forces, deciding one man
    should pay the price for pride,
another for disobedience,
    perhaps Athena would have said
of him, *It's not his time.*
    There is something he has left undone.
In hours and days of waiting,
    I watch monitors and charts,
learning the foreign language of ischemia,
    infarction,
ventricular fibrillation,
    plaque and platelet — that stop
the flow of vital oxygen and blood.

But other nouns
and verbs can block
    the pathways to the heart: moments
of our lives we let slip by
    through inattentive fingers,
smug confidence that
    makes us feel invincible.

I walk the park
   where flowers assail me like battalions
of wild color,
   hyperboles of purple, rose, magenta,
vermilion, violet, and gold.
   Life takes me by the neck
and shakes me hard,
   wake up, it's right here all around you.
This time Monet and Rumi
   send their messages to me.

The heart *is* a pump that needs to be addressed on a physical level, but our hearts are more than just pumps. A true physician is more than just a plumber, technician, or mechanic. We also have an emotional heart, a psychological heart, and a spiritual heart.

Our language reflects that understanding. We yearn for our sweethearts, not our sweetpumps. Poets and musicians and artists and writers and mystics throughout the ages have described those who have an open heart or a closed heart; a warm heart or a cold heart; a compassionate heart or an uncaring heart. Love heals. These are metaphors, a reflection of our deeper wisdom, not just figures of speech.

When I lecture at scientific meetings, hospitals, or medical schools, I always start by providing the scientific data as a way of establishing credibility. I show objective evidence from our randomized controlled trials that the progression of heart disease often can be reversed by changing lifestyle. *Then* I talk about what most interests me: the emotional, psychosocial, and spiritual dimensions of "opening your heart."

Afterward, I sometimes hear, "Gee, Dean, your lecture was really good until you got into that touchy-feely stuff."

Yet we *are* touchy-feely creatures. We are creatures of community. Those individuals, societies, and cultures who learned to take care of each other, to love each other, and to nurture relationships with each other during the past several hundred thousand years were more likely to survive than those who did not. Those people who did not learn to take care of each other often did not make it. In our culture, the idea of spending time taking care of each other and creating communities has become increasingly rare. Ignoring these ideas imperils our survival.

That which seems the most soft — love, intimacy, and meaning — is, in reality, the most powerful. This part of my work is the least well understood and yet perhaps the most important. There is a deep spiritual hunger in this country as we approach the end of the twentieth century and the beginning of a new millennium. There has been a radical shift in our society in the past fifty years, and we are only now beginning to appreciate what that really means.

The real epidemic in our culture is not only physical heart disease, but also what I call *emotional and spiritual heart disease* — that is, the profound feelings of loneliness, isolation, alienation, and depression that are so prevalent in our culture with the breakdown of the social structures that used to provide us with a sense of connection and community. It is, to me, a root of the illness, cynicism, and violence in our society.

Sometimes when I lecture I'll ask, "How many of you can say all four of these statements are true?"

- You live in the same neighborhood in which you were born and raised and most of your old neighbors are still there
- You've been going to the same church or synagogue for at least ten years and most of your fellow congregants from ten years ago are still there
- You've been at the same job for at least ten years and most of your coworkers from ten years ago are still there
- You have an extended family living nearby whom you see regularly

In an audience of three thousand people, maybe ten or twenty of them will raise their hands. And not just in San Francisco or New York or Los Angeles, but also in Ames, Iowa, or Omaha, Nebraska, the heart of the heartland. Fifty years ago, most would have been able to say yes.

Well, so what? What does this have to do with heart disease? What does this have to do with other illnesses? What does this have to do with health and healing? What does this have to do with much of anything?

It has everything to do with health and illness, with our survival as individuals and as a species. That is what this book is about.

Loneliness and isolation affect our health in several ways:

- They increase the likelihood that we may engage in behaviors like smoking and overeating that adversely affect our health and decrease the likelihood that we will make lifestyle choices that are life-enhancing rather than self-destructive
- They increase the likelihood of disease and premature death *from all causes* by 200 to 500 percent or more, independent of behaviors, through different mechanisms, many of which are not fully understood

- They keep us from fully experiencing the joy of everyday life

In short, *anything that promotes a sense of isolation often leads to illness and suffering. Anything that promotes a sense of love and intimacy, connection and community, is healing.* I will explore these themes in more detail in later chapters.

There is a good deal of suffering in our culture these days. It is very difficult to motivate people to make even simple changes in behavior like quitting smoking, changing diet, exercising, or even taking their medications when they feel depressed, lonely, and isolated. There are many, many ways of numbing pain, killing pain, distracting or distancing themselves from emotional pain. Some people smoke cigarettes. Others overeat, abuse drugs and alcohol, channel-surf, work too hard. Our culture provides us lots of ways to avoid pain — temporarily.

A well-known musician with heart disease came to see me. "I've been spending a lot of time at the track."

"That's good — exercise is important."

"No, not *that* track; the horses, man." Gambling is his way of distracting himself from his pain.

Suffering, in any of its many forms, can

be a doorway for real transformation, beyond just physical and behavioral changes. Why? Because change is not easy, at least at first. If you are suffering enough, and if the strategy for numbing the pain, distracting yourself from the pain, and killing the pain isn't working that well, then the idea of change begins to look more attractive.

You may say, in effect, "Well, it may be hard to change, but I'm in so much pain — almost anything is better than this. I will give your program a try." When people find how quickly they feel better, then the choices become clearer and, for many people, worth making. The reason for changing is reframed — people change not only to live longer, but also to live better.

Most physicians are not trained to deal with suffering as a doorway or as a catalyst for transformation. We are trained to view pain as an enemy and to kill the pain as quickly as possible. If somebody comes into the emergency room with a heart attack, we give them nitroglycerin. If that doesn't work, we are taught to go to morphine or Demerol or whatever it takes to kill the pain.

Not that we should seek out pain, but the pain is there for a reason. It says, "Hey! Listen up! Pay attention! You're doing something that's not in your best interest." Pain is a messenger. Pain is information. If we don't listen to it — if we just kill the pain without listening to the message and addressing the underlying problem — it's like clipping the wires to a fire alarm and going back to sleep without putting out the fire while the flames rage higher and your house burns down. You're not really dealing with the cause of the problem.

Healing and curing are not the same. Disease and illness are not the same. Pain and suffering are not the same.

Curing is when the physical disease gets measurably better. Healing is a process of becoming whole. Even the words *heal* and *whole* and *holy* come from the same root. Returning healing to medicine is like returning justice to law.

In my work with people who have heart disease, both healing and curing often occur. When the emotional heart and the spiritual heart begin to open, the physical heart often follows. In our research, my colleagues and I found a remarkable correlation between adherence to my program and changes in coronary artery blockages and blood flow to the heart. In other words, the more people changed, on average, the better they got. The amount of reversal of coronary artery disease was primarily a function neither of age nor disease severity but of how much patients changed their lifestyles.

Although most people got better, not everyone did. You can follow my program perfectly, but there are no guarantees that your heart disease will begin reversing. There is an element of mystery or destiny or luck or karma to all of this. *Healing may occur even when curing is not possible.* We can move closer to wholeness even when the physical illness does not improve. In the process of healing, you reach a place of wholeness and deep inner peace from which you can deal with illness with much less fear and suffering and much greater clarity and compassion. While curing is wonderful when it occurs, healing is often more meaningful because it takes you to a place of greater freedom from suffering.

Just as healing and curing are not the same, neither are pain and suffering. Pain is a physical process, the neural transmission of information to your brain when you injure yourself. Suffering is the perception of that experience. Even when pain cannot be modified, the experience — suffering — can be greatly reduced. Similarly, disease is the physical manifestation of biological dysfunction. Illness is your experience of that process and your relationship to it.

Victor Frankl was a physician and psychiatrist who was imprisoned during World War II in Auschwitz, a Nazi concentration camp. He wondered why some people survived and others did not. Some people who were relatively young and healthy seemed to give up and often died soon thereafter; others who were old, frail, and quite sick were able to survive and function despite overwhelming odds. He noticed that their survival was much less a factor of age or infirmity than their ability to find a sense of meaning in the midst of this horrible experience.

This sense of meaning in their lives was not necessarily religious or spiritual, although often it was. Some people wanted to live to bear witness; others for love — to help a parent or spouse or child who was there with them. Although the reason for each person may have been different, the deep sense of meaning that the reason provided enabled them to endure the most profound pain with much less suffering. The prison guards couldn't touch it or take it away. In short, the sense of meaning helped them survive.

Many patients have told me, "Having a heart attack was the best thing that ever happened to me." Part of the physical heart may remain damaged and scarred, yet their emotional and spiritual hearts may open in ways that transform the joy and meaning in their lives. Not everyone needs to have a heart attack for this to occur, but some people have told me that without having experienced a major traumatic event like that, it would have been unlikely for these other changes in their lives to have occurred. *Their suffering got their attention.*

Of course, I would never go up to someone and say, "Hey, isn't it great that you've had a heart attack!" If I did, the proper response would be a punch in the nose. Nevertheless, suffering of any kind can be a doorway for opening our hearts in ways that might not otherwise have occurred. Not that we look for suffering, but we can understand its alchemy and the possibilities for transformation when it happens.

Dr. Julia Rowlands is the head of psycho-oncology at Georgetown Medical School. When she interviews breast cancer patients, she has noted that if she took the word "cancer" out of their interviews and they just talked about what kind of change in life had taken place for them, that this often would sound like some extraordinarily positive experience. In other words, they often say things like "I've gotten in touch with my values and what's important to me in a way I haven't before." "It is much clearer to me what matters." "My relationships have gotten better or it's become more apparent to me which ones I shouldn't continue."

There is an enormous clarification process that tends to take place that often leads to healing. A recent guest editorial in the *Journal of the American Medical Association* by Dr. David Mumford, one of my mentors during medical school, was entitled, "Thank God I Have Cancer."[27] He described a patient who said:

> "David . . . let me tell you something. I've been imagining how it would be if my coming death were caused by a stroke, heart attack, or some other abrupt ending. When I do, I thank God I have cancer." He paused a moment and explained. "Without this extra time, I never would have known what love and tenderness are possible between people on this earth."

This is often where healing is the most profound, even when it is difficult to measure. This is often where healing is the most personally meaningful, even when it is difficult to describe.

Telling someone who is depressed, lonely, and isolated that they're going to live longer if they simply stop smoking, exercise, and eat a low-fat diet is not terribly motivating. Fewer than 50 percent of the people who were prescribed Mevacor, a cholesterol-lowering drug, are still taking it after just one year. Just one pill a day, and it doesn't have that many side effects.

Why? We take it for granted that people want to live longer, but many do not. After all, who wants to live longer if they're unhappy, depressed, and lonely?

When we address the deeper issues — the pain, loneliness, and isolation — then people are often much more willing to make lifestyle choices that are life-enhancing than ones that are self-destructive.

Many people in our culture walk around in varying degrees of chronic emotional pain. Some have told me that if they could just go to sleep and not wake up, that would be fine with them. They may not talk about this pain because they feel as if they have no one with whom they can talk openly and share these feelings — if they did, they wouldn't feel so lonely. Since they don't talk about their emotional pain with other people, it often seems they are alone in feeling this way; everyone else seems to have it all together. With such a perception, a person becomes even more lonely, more isolated, and more depressed.

Robert Reich was Secretary of Labor from 1993 to 1997. In a review of his book, the *New York Times* wrote:

> In Mr. Reich's Washington, everyone, including the author, wears a mask of self-assurance and competence in public. Privately, they are as befuddled and mistake-prone as everyone else, stumbling into success and failure alike.[28]

On the surface, it might seem that very successful people would have less emotional pain — but most of them do not. Trying to fill that void with success — whether measured in dollars, position, beauty, power, name, or fame — is like trying to quench a fire by pouring gasoline on it.

When people are unable to experience the feeling of connection and community in healing ways, they will often find it in ways that are dark and destructive. The powerful human need for intimacy, connection, and community can be harnessed for healing, as we have discussed, but also can be distorted in ways that may lead to disease, despair, and darkness.

This need for intimacy is so powerful that it may even override our basic survival instincts. Joining a gang is becoming a popular way of getting a sense of community and family, even if you have to rob or to kill somebody to join the gang. Joining a cult is another way. In Japan, a cult of people tried to poison the entire country. The members were, in many cases, the elite of the academic world in Japan. In San Diego, thirty-nine people chose to commit suicide together in 1997, many of whom already had undergone surgical castration in order to be part of that community. The need for a sense of community goes beyond us as individuals. Community can be developed in ways that bring us toward healing or, as these examples show, closer to suffering.

One way to have a sense of community is to form smaller and smaller tribes around the hatred of a common enemy. What we are often seeing around the world now is this balkanization and tribalization, the breakdown into smaller and smaller units based on seeing the differences between "us" and "them," the true believers and the heretics. Not only in Bosnia or in Chechnya, but also in the rise of political, religious, and social fundamentalism in all parts of the world. I imagine that one of the reasons why the movie *Independence Day* was so successful is that the entire world came together to fight the alien invaders, just as during the Gulf

War Americans huddled together to watch CNN as the war unfolded on television.

When we revert to tribes to find community based on having a common enemy, we fight those who are different from us. Ultimately, it is a false sense of community, because a tribe that is unified by anger, fear, and paranoia is likely to turn that suspicion on its own members until it breaks down further and further.

We can create communities and relationships that are based on love and intimacy rather than fear and hatred. We can learn from the suffering of others. Awareness is the first stage in healing.

Likewise, we can create a new model of medicine as we move into the next century that is more competent and cost-effective as well as being more caring and compassionate. In 1984, I founded the Preventive Medicine Research Institute, a nonprofit organization dedicated to research, education, and service. This institute has enabled me to bring together an extraordinary community of dedicated people who are highly accomplished and well trained *and* who are very nurturing and loving. While we do not always practice what we preach, all of us share the intention to model in our relationships with each other what we are trying to teach others.

Our work is based on the premise that addressing the underlying *causes* of a problem is ultimately more effective than addressing only its *symptoms*. In this context, efforts to contain medical costs that do not address the more fundamental lifestyle choices that determine *why* people become sick — rather than literally or figuratively bypassing them — inevitably result in painful choices. Our program of comprehensive lifestyle changes addresses not only behaviors like diet and lifestyle but also the underlying causes that often motivate these behaviors — including the lack of love and intimacy that so many people perceive in their lives.

For the past five years, we have conducted a demonstration project to learn if our program can be an alternative to coronary bypass surgery, angioplasty, and a lifetime of medications for selected people with severe coronary heart disease. We trained teams of nurses, physicians, dietitians, group support leaders, yoga/meditation teachers, chefs, exercise physiologists, and administrators in a very diverse group of hospitals across the country.

In the past, insurance companies have been reluctant to pay for lifestyle interventions because they were viewed as increasing costs in the short run for a possible savings years later. In the new model we are studying, every patient who can avoid surgery by changing lifestyle saves the insurance company tens of thousands of dollars *immediately* that otherwise may have been spent, not to mention sparing the patient the trauma of having his or her chest and leg cut open.

We found that most of the people who were eligible for surgery were able to avoid it by changing lifestyle, thereby saving thousands of dollars per patient. Mutual of Omaha was the first insurance company to cover our program; now, more than forty major insurance companies are covering it in the hospitals we have trained. They are finding it is good business to help patients open their hearts.

We are grateful that the Health Care Financing Administration is about to begin a similar demonstration project in these hospitals for Medicare patients. If we demonstrate similar adherence and cost savings in the Medicare population, then these practices may save billions of dollars per year. Medicare coverage is the primary determinant of medical practice and medical education in this country, because we physicians get trained to do what we get paid to do. If Medicare chooses to make this a defined benefit, then other insurance companies will likely follow their lead and also provide coverage for our program, thereby making it available to those who most need it.

This book chronicles my personal journey of exploration along with my experience as a physician and a scientist. For me, the most interesting books are ones in which the writer recreates his path for the reader, rather than acting like a guru coming down from the mountain to deliver a message. I usually find that the process of discovery is more interesting than the answers.

I have written this book from my own experience, as a researcher and from my inner life. The only person I'm trying to change is myself, and that's hard enough. Sections of this book are very self-revealing in order to share with you how I came to understand the healing power of love and intimacy — my loneliness and feelings of isolation earlier in life, the mistakes I have made, and some of what I have learned along the way. I hope you will find at least some of it useful.

Chapter 2 of this book is a systematic review of the science supporting the important role of social support and intimacy in health and illness. Science gives us knowledge, but we also need wisdom; chapter 3 describes in very personal and self-disclosing terms my own struggles with intimacy in my personal life and what I am learning from that process. Chapter 4 describes some powerful strategies and techniques for enhancing intimacy that I have found to be helpful in my own life and in working with others. Chapter 5 gives a meaningful example from my clinical experience.

The scientific evidence I review in chapter 2 leaves little doubt that love and intimacy are powerful determinants of our health and survival. *Why* they have such an impact remains somewhat a mystery. In chapter 6, I have interviewed an eclectic group of leading authorities from disparate backgrounds — eminent scientists, psychologists, physicians, healers, theologians, authors, and others — each of whom brings a unique perspective to answering the question of why love and intimacy have such a powerful effect on our health and survival.

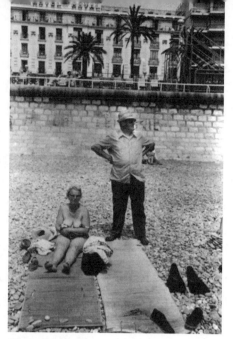

Copenhagen, 1974

2

The Scientific Basis
for the
Healing Power of Intimacy

The healing power of love and relationships has been documented in an increasing number of well-designed scientific studies involving hundreds of thousands of people throughout the world. I will review a number of these studies in the following pages as a way of demonstrating the scientific basis for the healing power of love and intimacy, community and communion. *They matter.* Loneliness hurts.

Awareness is the first step in healing, for individuals as well as society. Sometimes the brain needs to be satisfied before the heart begins to open. For many researchers, "love" might as well be a four-letter word, and "an open heart" is what happens during coronary bypass surgery. Instead, scientists tend to use such other terms as social support, intimacy, hostility, depression, anger, cynicism, and so on. Remember the story of the blind men and the elephant? Every person had a different perspective on what the elephant looked like. Each term is a different facet of an overall truth.

I believe these different terms and perspectives share a common root: love. As I use these terms in this book — social support, connection, community, and related ideas — all relate to a common theme. When you feel loved, nurtured, cared for, supported, and intimate, you are much more likely to be happier and healthier. You have a much lower risk of getting sick and, if you do, a much greater chance of surviving.

During the past twenty years of conducting research, I have become increasingly aware of the importance of love and intimacy and knew there were many studies documenting their power. Not until I systematically reviewed the scientific literature for this book did I realize just how extensive and rich is this field of study.

"Does Your Wife Show You Her Love?"

While some studies measure the *number* or *structure* of social relationships, I believe that it is your perception of the *quality* of those relationships — how you feel about them — that is most important.[1] As two distinguished researchers wrote recently, "Social support reflects loving and caring relationships in people's lives. . . . Simple ratings of feeling loved may be as effective, if not more effective, in assessing social support than more comprehensive instruments that quantify network size, structure, and function."[2]

At Yale, for example, scientists studied 119 men and 40 women who were undergoing coronary angiography, an X-ray movie that shows the degree of blockages in coronary arteries. Those who felt the most loved and supported had substantially less blockage in the arteries of their hearts.[3] The researchers found that feelings of being loved and emotionally supported were more important predictors of the severity of coronary artery blockages than was the number of relationships a person had. Equally important, this effect was independent of diet, smoking, exercise, cholesterol, family history (genetics), and other standard risk factors.

A study of 131 women in Sweden also found that the availability of deep emotional relationships was associated with less coronary artery blockage as measured by computer-analyzed coronary angiography. As in the Yale study, this finding remained true even when controlling for age, hypertension, smoking, diabetes, cholesterol, educational level, menopausal status, and other factors that might have influenced the extent of disease.[4]

Similarly, researchers from Case Western Reserve University in Cleveland studied almost ten thousand married men with no prior history of angina (chest pain). Men who had high levels of risk factors such as elevated cholesterol, high blood pressure, age, diabetes, and electrocardiogram abnormalities were over twenty times more likely to develop new angina during the next five years.

However, those who answered "yes" to the simple question, "Does your wife show you her love?" had significantly less angina even when they had high levels of these risk factors. Men who had these risk factors but did not have a wife who showed her love had substantially increased angina — almost twice as much. The greater the cholesterol and blood pressure and the greater the anxiety and stress, the more important was the love of the spouse in buffering against these harmful effects.

As the researchers wrote, "The wife's love and support is an important balancing factor which apparently reduces the risk of angina pectoris even in the presence of high risk factors."[5] The researchers also found that those men who also had anxiety and family problems, especially conflicts with their wives and children, had even more chest pain. They went on to conclude:

The implications of these findings for clinicians lie in two directions. In the one, preventive measures, like anti-smoking, reducing cholesterol and blood pressure levels and weight, will probably help to reduce the incidence of myocardial infarction and, to a lesser extent, angina pectoris. But in the other, no matter how well this is done, the major sources of risk for angina pectoris will be missed, unless it is accompanied by a detailed investigation of the subject's personal, family, and occupational life situations. . . . It again stresses the often-mentioned need for, but rarely performed, coverage of the physical, emotional, and social aspects of the patient's life in order to prevent, delay, or diminish his angina pectoris.

In other words, although diet, blood pressure, and other risk factors play an important role in developing heart disease and angina, *these forces can be significantly moderated by a loving relationship.* Although researchers did not study women or same-sex couples with heart disease, my clinical experience with them has been similar.

In a related study, these researchers studied almost 8,500 men with no history or symptoms of duodenal ulcer. These men were given questionnaires before they developed ulcers, so their responses were not influenced by knowing they had this disease.

Over the next five years, 254 of these men developed ulcers. Those who had reported a low level of perceived love and support from their wives when they entered the study had over *twice as many* ulcers as the other men. Those men who answered, "My wife does not love me" had almost *three times* as many ulcers as those who said their wives showed their love and support. This factor was more strongly associated with ulcers than smoking, age, blood pressure, job stress, or other factors. Men who also had anxiety and family problems had more ulcers.[6]

The current thinking in medicine is that many ulcers are caused by infection with a bacterium, *Helicobacter pylori.* Nevertheless, men who felt loved by their wives were somehow protected to a great degree even from getting ulcers even though presumably infected with this organism. As we will see later, infection may be a *necessary* but not *sufficient* prerequisite for illness to manifest when a person feels love and support.

Who Do You Love?

How do scientists measure love and support? It is easier just to measure the *number* of social relationships than a person's perceptions of the *quality* of those relationships.[7] In one study, for example, the researchers measured the *number* of social relationships by asking about:

The number of people you meet during an ordinary week

The number of people with whom you share interests

The number of friends who at any time would come and visit your home and you wouldn't be embarrassed if it were messy

The number of friends or family members with whom you can talk frankly

The investigators measured the *quality* of those emotional relationships by asking if you have:

Someone special, whom you can lean on

Someone who feels very close to you

Someone to share feelings with

Someone to confide in

Someone to hold and comfort you

Someone at home who really appreciates what you do for him/her

The researchers found that both the number and the quality of relationships were important.[8] Of course, having a large number of destructive relationships is not desirable, so the *quality* of the relationships — how loving and supportive they are — is more important than the *number* of those relationships.

Another group of scientists defined social support in three categories.[9] *Emotional support* involves the verbal and nonverbal communication of caring and concern — that you are valued and loved and have the opportunity for intimacy. Emotional support can help provide a sense of purpose, meaning, and belonging. *Informational support* gives you access to information, advice, appraisal, and guidance from others. *Instrumental support* gives you access to material or physical assistance, such as access to transportation, money, or assistance with chores.[10] While these distinctions may be useful for designing research studies, I think these categories are simply subsets of a more basic one: Do you feel loved and cared for?

Other researchers who measure social support might ask questions like these:

> If you became ill, is there a friend who would drive you to the hospital or would you have to take a taxi or ambulance?
>
> If you were broke, is there a friend who would loan you money?
>
> If you were sick, is there a friend who would help take care of your children until you felt better?

In other words, do you have anyone who really cares for you? Who feels close to you? Who loves you? Who wants to help you? In whom you can confide?

If the answers are "no," you may have *three to five times* higher risk of premature death and disease from all causes — or even higher, according to some studies. These include increased risk of heart attack, stroke, infectious diseases, many types of cancer, allergies, arthritis, tuberculosis, autoimmune diseases, low birth weight and low Apgar scores, alcoholism, drug abuse, suicide, and so on. This reduction in premature death was found both in people who were healthy and in those who were unhealthy at the start of these studies.[11] Also, people are much more likely to choose life-enhancing behaviors rather than self-destructive ones when they feel loved and cared for.[12, 13]

What is also important in a number of studies is not only how much you *get* but also how much you *give*. Giving and receiving love and intimacy are healing for both the giver and for the recipient.

In one study of more than seven hundred elderly adults, for example, the effects of aging had more to do with what they contributed to their social support network than what they received from it. The more love and support they offered, the more they benefited themselves.[14] One of the simplest and most elegant definitions of social support is this: "Social support is defined as information leading the subject to believe that he is cared for and loved, esteemed, and a member of a network of mutual obligations."

Put in another way, anything that promotes feelings of love and intimacy is healing; anything that promotes isolation, separation, loneliness, loss, hostility, anger, cynicism, depression, alienation, and related feelings often leads to suffering, disease, and premature death from all causes. While the evidence on the relationship of psychosocial factors to illness is controversial,[15] most scientific studies have demonstrated the extraordinarily powerful role of love and relationships in determining health and illness.

Lonely or Alone

I want to distinguish between feeling lonely and being alone. You can feel lonely while walking down the street in New York City surrounded by thousands of people. You can be filled with love and feelings of interconnectedness while meditating or praying alone in church, synagogue, or a mountaintop. Love and interconnectedness come in many forms — with other people, of course, but also with a pet, or with a spiritual force, whatever name we give to that. It is the *experience* and the *perception* of loneliness that seem to determine its effects on our health and well-being. In a very real sense, perception *is* reality.

Similarly, *community* used to refer just to the people in the neighborhood where you live. There was a sense of familiarity, safety, comfort; a place where you knew and were known by most of the other people there. Now, many people barely know — if at all — the person in the apartment or house next door.

New communities and new relationships are forming. The perception of community — the feelings of familiarity, safety, and comfort — now may transcend the neighborhood and involve a network of people throughout the country. These "virtual communities" come in many different forms but may serve a similar purpose.[16] These include E-mail, chat rooms in on-line services, Internet support groups, and so on.

When I reviewed the scientific literature, I was amazed to find what a powerful difference love and relationships make on the incidence of disease and premature death from virtually *all* causes. It may be hard to believe that something as simple as talking with friends, feeling close to your parents, sharing feelings openly, or making yourself vulnerable to others in order to enhance intimacy can make such a powerful difference in your health and well-being, but study after study indicates that they often do. It's easy to make fun of these ideas — talking about your feelings in a group, opening your heart to others, practicing yoga, meditation, or prayer to rediscover inner sources of peace, joy, and well-being — but look at what a powerful difference they can make in our survival!

What's Love Got to Do with It?

The idea that one factor like social support can affect disease and death from virtually *all* causes is at odds with one of the most fundamental precepts of modern medicine: Koch's Postulate. In the nineteenth century, the German physician Robert Koch won the Nobel Prize for being one of the first to identify a specific agent (the tubercle bacillus) as the cause of a specific illness (tuberculosis). According to Koch, and later to the French scientist Louis Pasteur, who developed the germ theory, an organism is proven to cause a disease if you find it in animals or people who have the disease and if you inject it into animals or humans and can cause the disease. Diseases were caused by a single microbe and thus treatment should be directed at eradicating this microorganism. What's love got to do with it?

The problem with Koch's Postulate is that most people are not exposed to bacteria or viruses by injecting them (intravenous drug users being a notable exception). Bacteria, viruses, and other microorganisms must first penetrate through our immune, neuro-endocrine and other defense systems. As I will document later in this chapter, these defenses are enhanced and buffered by love and relationships. Not everyone exposed to bacteria and viruses becomes ill — otherwise, doctors and nurses who take care of patients would be sick all the time.

Even Pasteur changed his thinking later in life and believed that germs were only part of the picture and that other factors usually played an even more important role. According to legend, Pasteur said on his deathbed, *"Le germe n'est rien, c'est le terrain qui est tout"* ("The microbe is nothing, the soil is everything").[17]

In other words, exposure to bacteria, viruses, and other pathogens may be *necessary* but not *sufficient* to cause illness. For example, most people who test positive for being infected with the tubercle bacillus never develop tuberculosis. Most people who are infected with influenza viruses do not get the flu.

I cite a number of studies in this chapter that demonstrate that love and relationships are protective. They enhance our immune function and strengthen our resistance to disease. To use Pasteur's metaphor, loneliness and isolation help create a fertile soil for microbes to grow.

Prior to the discovery of the tubercle bacillus, the causes of tuberculosis were thought to be a combination of weather, emotional depression, and bad genes. When the bacillus was discovered, most of the attention focused on controlling its spread and developing drugs that could kill the bacillus while neglecting the psychosocial factors that help create a home for it. Now, we understand that treating the organism with drugs *and* addressing the psychosocial factors are important. For example, more than forty years ago, it was noted that the highest rates of tuberculosis are in isolated people with little social support, even when they live in wealthy neighborhoods.[18]

Similarly, how much cholesterol ends up in your arteries is only partly a function of how much fat and cholesterol you consume.

How your body metabolizes cholesterol and the likelihood of a heart attack or sudden cardiac death are also affected by love and relationships.

Dr. Lisa Berkman has been one of the leading scientists in exploring the role of social factors in health. She is now chair and professor of the department of health and social behavior and professor of epidemiology at the Harvard School of Public Health. In a recent journal article, she described the resistance she encountered, during her doctoral comprehensive examinations in 1975, to the idea that social factors might influence a broad range of disease outcomes. Here is an edited excerpt:

> I offered the opinion that social support and networks influence many disease outcomes because these social conditions influence susceptibility to disease in general. I went on to add some hypothetical pathways involving neuroendocrine regulation and potential immune responses, which in turn might influence diseases of an infectious nature and cancer and heart disease.
>
> At that point, the senior member of this committee proclaimed, "Over the last 150 years of medical research from

Pasteur and Koch onward, research has proceeded successfully along the lines of identifying one cause of one disease, with the theory of disease specificity being one of the major advances in our thinking over the last century." He went on to question whether we should invoke such vague concepts as "social forces." With more evidence than was available twenty years ago, I would like to respond to this issue today the way I responded to it then — with a "yes."[19]

The Harvard Mastery of Stress Study

One of the most interesting and powerful examples of how loving relationships may affect susceptibility to disease in general was a study of Harvard students by Drs. Stanley King, Harry Russek, Gary Schwartz, Linda Russek, and others.[20, 21] In the early 1950s, 126 healthy men were randomly chosen from the Harvard classes of 1952 to 1954 and given questionnaires to measure how they felt about their parents.

In the first test, students were asked,

Would you describe your relationship to your mother and to your father as [check one]:

Very close
Warm and friendly
Tolerant
Strained and cold

The choices were coded from 4 (very close) to 1 (strained and cold).

Thirty-five years later, medical records were obtained on these participants and detailed medical and psychological histories were conducted. What they found was quite amazing: 91 percent of participants who did not perceive themselves to have had a warm relationship with their mothers thirty-five years earlier had serious diagnosed diseases in midlife (including coronary artery disease, high blood pressure, duodenal ulcer, and alcoholism), as compared to only 45 percent of those who perceived themselves to have had a warm relationship with their mothers. Similarly, 82 percent of participants who had low warmth and closeness scores with their fathers had diagnosed diseases in midlife compared with only 50 percent of those who had high warmth and closeness scores with their fathers.

The effects of feeling warmth and closeness with mothers and fathers appeared to be additive. *All* (100 percent) of the participants who rated both their mothers and fathers low in warmth and closeness thirty-five years earlier had diseases diagnosed in midlife. Only 47 percent of those who rated both their fathers and mothers high in warmth and closeness had diagnosed diseases in midlife. The other two groups were intermediate. Seventy-five percent of those who rated their mother high but their father low in warmth and closeness had diagnosed diseases in midlife, and 83 percent of those who rated their father high but their mother low in warmth and closeness had diagnosed diseases in midlife.

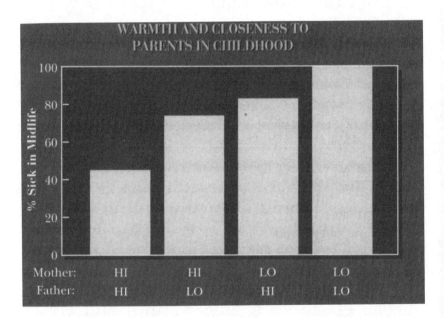

The researchers wrote, "The perception of love itself . . . may turn out to be a core biopsychosocial-spiritual buffer, reducing the negative impact of stressors and pathogens and promoting immune function and healing."

They also looked at their data in a slightly different way. These students were asked, "What kind of person is your mother?" and "What kind of person is your father?" The researchers simply counted the number of positive or negative words the students used in describing their parents.

They found that the number of positive descriptions while in college was a significant predictor of their future health and illness in midlife. Although the words provided by the students covered many facets of love and caring, a simple score reflecting the total number of positive words predicted future health and illness thirty-five years later.

The relationship of these descriptions of parental love and caring to future health was independent of family history of illness, smoking, emotional stress, subsequent death or divorce of parents, and the students' marital history. Also, students who were subsequently sick in midlife used a larger total number of negative words to describe their parents when they were in college.[22]

When these researchers combined these two measures — the ratings of warmth and closeness with parents in college and the number of positive descriptions when asked, "What kind of person is your mother and your father?" — they found *95 percent of subjects who used few positive words and also rated their parents low in parental caring had diseases diagnosed in midlife, whereas only 29 percent of subjects who used many positive words and also rated their parents high in parental caring had diseases diagnosed in midlife.*

Of course, saying negative words does not cause illness. These words reflect our perceptions of love and relationship and these perceptions, in turn, profoundly affect our health and survival.

These researchers also found that the perception of parental caring was additive with other risk factors, such as one's coping style under stress. They found that the combination of low perception of parental caring and the experience of severe anxiety assessed during college was additive. Only 24 percent of students with high positive perceptions of parental caring and low anxiety during college became sick in midlife, whereas 94 percent of those with low positive perceptions of parental caring and severe anxiety during college were sick in midlife.

The Johns Hopkins Study

In a related study, researchers at the Johns Hopkins Medical School tested and followed more than 1,100 male medical students in the 1940s. They were examining the hypothesis — that is, they wondered — if the quality of human relationships might be a factor in the development of cancer.[23]

The researchers used a questionnaire called the "Closeness to Parents Scale" to assess the quality of the students' relationships with their parents. At the time of this ques-

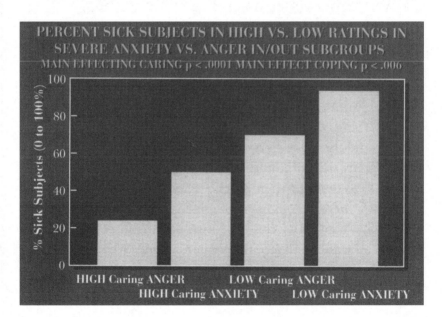

tionnaire, as in the Harvard study described above, all of these students were healthy.

Medical students who subsequently developed cancer were more likely to have described a lack of closeness with their parents than their healthy classmates when they were tested up to *fifty years earlier*.[24] They found that the predictive value of this test did not diminish over time and was not explained by other known risk factors, such as smoking, drinking, or radiation exposure. They learned that the best predictor of who would get cancer decades later was the closeness of father-son relationships earlier in life.

They also found that those physicians who eventually committed suicide, had to be hospitalized for mental illness, or developed malignant tumors had suffered more from loneliness and had greater interpersonal difficulties one to fifty years earlier.[25] In a separate questionnaire, they found less satisfactory relationships among medical students who later developed cancer when compared with the other students at that time.[26]

The Durkheim Study

One of the first studies of the power of social support was in 1897 by the French sociologist Emile Durkheim. In his classic study, he noted that while suicide is one of the most individual acts, suicide rates varied among different groups and time periods. To explain this difference, Durkheim's research led him to conclude that the major factor affecting suicide rates was the degree of social integration of groups. He found that the extent to which an individual is integrated into group life determined whether he would be likely to commit suicide.[27] Durkheim also found that unmarried men and women were more likely to commit suicide than those who are married.[28]

The Scotland Study

In the 1950s, Dr. David Kissen and colleagues in Scotland studied men who entered the hospital with symptoms of chest discomfort, before they learned that they had cancer. Those who were subsequently diagnosed as having lung cancer had experienced significantly more difficulties much earlier in life (such as the death of one or both parents) than those who were found to have more benign diagnoses.[29] The researchers also found that those who were diagnosed with lung cancer tended to have more disturbed interpersonal relationships and had particular difficulty in expressing their emotions, especially those involving intimate relationships with their spouse or friends.[30]

Even Better

Did you come from a family where you want to reach out and touch someone? Or is long distance not only the next best thing to being there — it's even better? How can a relationship with parents decades earlier affect whether or not someone gets heart disease, cancer, or other causes of premature death and disability later in life? Does that mean a person who did not have an emotionally warm relationship with one or both parents or whose parents died early in life is doomed to early death and disease?

Not necessarily. We can't change what happened to us in our childhood or adolescence, but we do not need to do so. I believe that it is the *ongoing pattern of relating to others* that is most important, not a particular event that happened much earlier in life.

According to Drs. Russek and Schwartz, "The perception of parental love and caring may be a powerful predictor of future health because parental love and caring involves and integrates so many potential mechanisms."[31] These include:

- nutrition, stress, and loving energy before and after birth
- healthy and unhealthy behaviors developed during childhood
- coping styles such as anxiety, anger, hostility, depression, optimism, and self-esteem
- choice and stability of relationships and friendships
- the presence and support of parents in one's adult life
- spiritual values and practices.

An important reason why early relationships are so predictive of later illness is that these patterns of relating do not change very much in most people over time. As I described in chapter 1, change is not easy. Modifying such behaviors as diet, exercise, and smoking is hard enough. Changing our ongoing pattern of relating to others is even more difficult.

I know this as a scientist and from my clinical work with patients. I also know this from understanding how hard it has been for me to make fundamental changes in my own patterns of relating. As I began to realize the healing power of love and relationship, I began to devote more of my time and energy to working on my own wounded areas and helping the patients who came to me to do the same. I will describe this process later in this book.

In animals as well as in humans, resistance to a wide variety of diseases including malaria, cancer, and tuberculosis as well as premature death can be significantly changed by early life experiences. Dr. Robert Ader defined a new field, "psychoneuroimmunology," by studying the effects of social factors on the immune system of animals.[32, 33]

Opening Your Heart

Parents are usually the most important source of love, social support, and intimacy early in life. Psychotherapists sometimes call this "object relations" — that is, people often develop patterns of relating as adults that are not so different from how they learned to relate as children. If you grew up in a family in which love, nurturing, and intimacy are in short supply, then you are more likely to view your current relationships with mistrust and suspicion. If your family experiences were filled with love and caring, then you are more likely to be open and trusting in your ongoing relationships.

It is particularly difficult for us to develop intimate and loving relationships if we grew up in a family in which intimacy was dangerous because of emotional, physical, or sexual abuse.[34] The heart develops a particularly strong armor to protect and defend itself, but the same emotional defenses that protect us can also isolate us if they always remain up, if nowhere and no one feels safe enough for us to let down our walls. When I use the term "opening your heart," I mean your willingness to allow yourself to be open and vulnerable to another person.

We can only be intimate to the degree that we are willing to be open and vulnerable. When people are abused by those who are supposed to nurture and protect them, especially in childhood, it is not surprising that they will have a more difficult time trusting others later in life.

As one group of researchers wrote, "Those most in need of the support provided by a good marriage may not be able to benefit from it because the ability to form close relationships may itself be impaired by earlier adversity. . . . A negative bonding experience [with parents] may result in the failure to acquire a true sense of self and resilient self-esteem, attributes promoting coping in later life. This may result in the avoidance of close relationships for fear of intimacy, failure, and/or rejection."[35]

It doesn't have to be that way. Old wounds can begin to heal.

According to some researchers, an intimate, loving relationship as an adult can offset many of the harmful effects of childhood adversity and parental deprivation. Whom you choose to be with in a relationship — and how you relate to that person — can either help overcome adverse childhood experiences or reinforce them.[36] I have experienced both types of relationships, and I will write more about these experiences in the next chapter.

While the most extreme forms of childhood deprivation can be difficult to overcome, others can change. According to a recent review article, "Those exposed to extreme deficits in early parental care appear more likely to associate with an uncaring intimate partner (if a relationship is established at all). However, any initial vulnerability established under less extreme difficulties in the parent-child relationship appears capable of being modified by later relational experiences with intimate partners and with significant others."[37]

The Roseto Study

One of the earliest and most important studies recognizing the power of love and relationships to modify the harmful effects of otherwise unhealthful behaviors was in Roseto, Pennsylvania, an Italian-American town in eastern Pennsylvania. Roseto has been studied intensively for over fifty years.

The population of Roseto was found to have had a strikingly low mortality rate from heart attacks during the first thirty years it was studied when compared to Bangor, an immediately adjacent town, and Nazareth, another nearby community. The risk factors for heart disease such as smoking, high-fat diet, diabetes, and so on were at least as prevalent in Roseto as in Bangor and Nazareth. All three communities were served by the same hospital facilities, water supply, and physicians.

Why was the incidence of heart attacks so much lower in Roseto? At the time, Roseto, which had been settled by immigrants from a town in southern Italy in 1882, still displayed a high level of ethnic and social homogeneity, close family ties, and cohesive community relationships. The researchers wondered if Roseto's stable structure, its emphasis on family cohesion, and the supportive nature of the community may have been protective against heart attacks and conducive to longevity.

They were right: In the late 1960s and early 1970s, Roseto shifted from three-generation households with strong commitments to religion, relationships, and traditional values and practices to a less cohesive, fragmented, and isolated community. This loosening of family ties and weakening of the community in Roseto was accompanied by a substantial increase in death due to heart attacks. During this time, the mortality rate rose to the same level as that of the neighboring communities.[38]

The Roseto study demonstrated the importance of relationships. As the researchers wrote, "Those with the conventional risk factors are more likely to develop myocardial infarction [heart attacks] than are those without the risk factors, but an even larger proportion of the population may have the risk factors and not succumb to myocardial infarction over a period of nearly three decades" if they are protected by a strong sense of connection and community.[39]

Between 1979 and 1994, eight large-scale community-based studies were conducted to examine the relationship between social isolation and death and disease from all causes.

Although there was a lot of variation in these communities — from California to Eastern Finland, from Georgia to Sweden — as well as differences in how social support and social isolation were measured, these studies showed remarkably consistent results. *Those who were socially isolated had at least two to five times the risk of premature death from all causes when compared to those who had a strong sense of connection and community.* Let's examine some of these.

The Alameda County Study

In 1965, Dr. Berkman and her colleagues at the California Department of Health Services began studying almost seven thousand men and women living in Alameda County, located near San Francisco. They found that those who lacked social and community ties (contact with friends and relatives, marriage, and church and group membership) were 1.9 to 3.1 times more likely to die during the nine-year follow-up period from 1965 to 1974.[40]

This association between social and community ties and premature death was found to be independent of and a more powerful predictor of health and longevity than age, gender, race, socioeconomic status, self-reported physical health status, and health practices such as smoking, alcoholic beverage consumption, overeating, physical activity, and utilization of preventive health services as well as a cumulative index of health practices. Those who lacked social ties were at increased risk of dying from coronary heart disease, stroke, cancer, respiratory diseases, gastrointestinal diseases, and all other causes of death.[41]

The researchers continued to follow these people for eight more years (a total of seventeen years). They found the same results: Those with the strongest social ties had dramatically lower rates of disease and premature death than those who felt isolated and alone.

Those with close social ties and unhealthful lifestyles actually lived longer than those with poor social ties but more healthful behaviors. Not surprisingly, those who lived the longest had both close social ties *and* healthful behaviors.[42]

Women who were socially isolated or who even just *felt* they were isolated had a significantly elevated risk of dying of cancer of all sites as well as from smoking-related cancers. Men with few social connections showed significantly poorer cancer survival rates.[43] The absence of close ties and perceived sources of emotional support was associated significantly with an increased breast cancer death rate.

The relationship between social ties, stage of disease, and survival was analyzed in a subset of 525 black and 486 white women in Alameda County with newly diagnosed breast cancer. The absence of close ties and perceived sources of emotional support was associated with a significantly increased breast cancer death rate. Both black women and white women reporting few sources of emotional support had almost twice the death rate from breast cancer during the five-year period of follow-up.[44]

Another group of researchers studied 283 women with breast cancer who were diagnosed between 1958 and 1960. At the time of diagnosis, these women were interviewed about the amount of stress and social support present in the five-year period preceding their diagnosis. Twenty years later, these interviews helped predict survival: Social stress decreased and social involvement increased the length of time these women survived.[45]

The Tecumseh Study

In the Tecumseh Community Health Study, almost three thousand men and women were studied for nine to twelve years. After adjustments for age and a variety of risk factors for mortality, men reporting higher levels of social relationships and activities were significantly less likely to die during the follow-up period. Relationships included the number of friends, how close they felt to their relatives, group activities, and so on. When these social relationships were broken or decreased, disease rates increased *two to three times* as much during the succeeding ten-to-twelve-year period, including heart disease, strokes, cancer, arthritis, and lung diseases. As in the Alameda County study, these results were not related to age, occupation, or health status, including blood pressure, cholesterol, electrocardiogram results, and so on.[46]

The Swedish Studies

In Sweden, more than seventeen thousand men and women between the ages of twenty-nine and seventy-four were followed for six years. Those who were the most lonely and isolated had almost *four times* the risk of dying prematurely during this period. Controlling for age and sex, age and educational level, age and employment status, age and immigrant status, age and smoking, age and exercise habits, and age and chronic disease at interview left the relative risk virtually unchanged.[47] In another study of elderly men living in Sweden, those who had a low availability of emotional support or who lived alone had more than *double* the premature death rate of the other men, even after controlling for other factors that influence disease.[48]

The Beta-Blocker Heart Attack Trial

Researchers in the "Beta-Blocker Heart Attack Trial" interviewed more than 2,300 men who had survived a heart attack. Those who were classified as being socially isolated and having a high degree of life stress had more than *four times* the risk of death as men who had low levels of both stress and isolation, even when controlling for other prognostic factors such as genetics, smoking, diet, alcohol, exercise, weight, and so on. The increase in risk associated with stress and social isolation applied both to total deaths and to sudden cardiac deaths.[49] These psychosocial effects had a much more powerful effect on premature deaths than did the beta-blocker drug being tested, even though beta-blockers are widely prescribed by many cardiologists whereas psychosocial factors are often ignored by them.

The Finland Study

The power of social support also was seen clearly in the North Karelia Project in Finland. More than thirteen thousand people were studied. Over five to nine years, those men who were socially isolated had an increased risk of death *two to three times* higher than those who had the greatest sense of social connection and community. These results were found even when there was extensive adjustment for traditional cardiovascular risk factors such as cholesterol, age, smoking, serum cholesterol, and blood pressure.[50]

The Evans County Study

Similar results were found in a study in Evans County, Georgia, of over two thousand people.[51] Using a similar questionnaire to the Alameda County study, researchers found that marriage, contacts with extended family and friends, church membership, and group affiliations predicted mortality in men after eleven to thirteen years, even after adjusting for other factors. No relationship was found in women, but they had very low mortality rates, which may have made it more difficult to detect a relationship. Also, reductions in social connections were prospectively associated with increased risk of death from coronary heart disease during the following nine years.[52]

The Three Communities Study

In another study, identical measures of social connections were obtained from three community-based groups whose members were aged sixty-five and over from East Boston, Massachusetts; New Haven, Connecticut; and two rural counties in Iowa to see if social isolation increases mortality risks for older men and women. After five years in all three communities, those with no social ties had a *two to three times* increased risk of mortality compared to those with at least four social ties.[53]

That's What Friends Are For

Many studies have shown that married people live longer, with lower mortality for almost every major cause of death, than those who are single, separated, widowed, or divorced.[54] Married people have both a lower incidence of disease and better survival after diagnosis.[55]

The percentage of persons surviving at least five years after diagnosis of cancer is greater for married than unmarried persons in almost every category of age, gender, and stage. Even after controlling for stage at diagnosis and treatment, married people have better survival. As the authors wrote, "The results of this study do not allow us to determine if the beneficial effect of being married on survival with cancer is mediated via social, psychological, economic, or other forces, or whether, as may be likely, all are involved. We emphasize, however, the practical consequences of our findings. The decreases in survival associated with being unmarried are not trivial and apply to a large population at risk."[56]

For example, Dr. Redford Williams and his colleagues at Duke studied almost fourteen hundred men and women who underwent coronary angiography and were found to have had at least one severely blocked coronary artery. After five years, men and women who were unmarried and who did not have a close confidant — someone to talk with on a regular basis — were over *three times* as likely to have died than those who were married, had a confidant, or both.

After five years, fifty percent of those who

were unmarried and who did not have a confidant were dead. Again, these differences were independent of any other known medical prognostic risk factors, including number and severity of blocked coronary arteries, left ventricular function, smoking, cholesterol, exercise, and so on.[57]

Of interest in that study was that even those who were married but did not have a confidant did better than those who were unmarried and had no confidant. Just living with someone is better than being isolated, at least according to this study.

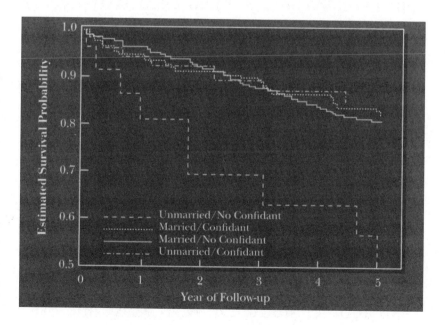

Another study in Baltimore found similar results. Almost nine hundred married men and women who experienced an acute heart attack had a significantly better survival prospect, both in the hospital and even ten years after discharge, independent of other factors.[58] A study of over two hundred men in Sweden who suffered a heart attack found that being single significantly increased the risk of death both from heart disease and from all causes more than eight years later.[59]

In Durham, North Carolina, Dr. D. G. Blazer studied the effects of social support on 331 men and women aged sixty-five or over. Those who perceived their social support as impaired were *386 percent* more likely to die prematurely after only thirty months. Even after Dr. Blazer controlled for other potentially confounding influences — including age, sex, race, economic status, physical health status, self-care capacity, depressive symptoms, cognitive functioning, stressful life events, and cigarette smoking — those who perceived their social support as impaired were 340 percent more likely to die prematurely from all causes.[60]

In another study, Dr. R. B. Case and others conducted a study to find out if people who had recently suffered a heart attack and who lived alone were at higher risk of having another heart attack or dying than those who lived with one or more other people.

The answer was clearly *yes:* Those who lived alone had almost *twice as many* heart attacks and deaths after six months as the others. The risk remained similar for the next one to four years and was independent of age, gender, the severity of damage to the heart, irregular heartbeats, drug treatments, or subsequent angioplasty or bypass surgery. As the authors wrote, "Recurrent cardiac event rate and cardiac death rate were both much lower in those who lived with others, suggesting that living with others, at least in this situation, provides some sort of protective effect."[61]

Researchers in Amsterdam interviewed over 2,800 Dutch citizens, fifty-five to eighty-five years of age. The interviews helped determine levels of loneliness as well as individual perceptions of the emotional support available from family and friends. The researchers then tracked deaths among the study subjects for almost two and a half years. They discovered that older persons who perceived themselves as surrounded by a loving, supportive circle of friends "decreased their likelihood of dying by approximately half" when compared with individuals who reported feelings of emotional isolation. Those with the highest self-reported feelings of loneliness had nearly *double* the death rate of those who said they felt emotionally connected to others.[62]

In another study, researchers in Vermont found that a perceived lack of support from others was "a significant predictor of death and greater functional deterioration" in heart disease patients. The study focused on a group of 820 Canadian heart disease patients, each of whom was questioned as to their perceived need for help with the activities of daily living, such as bathing and preparing food. The health progress of those individuals was then followed for one year. Patient perceptions of unmet needs seemed strongly linked to an increased risk for death.

Compared with the patients who said they had "no perceived need" of outside support, those who acknowledged they needed "more help" had over *triple* the risk of dying during the one-year period of the study. Study participants requiring "much more help" had a *six and one-half times greater risk of dying* than those most satisfied with the support system around them. The researchers noted that "individuals who were single or lived alone were less likely to perceive adequate tangible support" than those who lived with others.[63]

Dr. L. F. Berkman and her colleagues examined the survival of elderly men and women hospitalized for an acute heart attack who had emotional support compared with those patients who lacked such emotional support. More than *three times* as many men and women who had no source of emotional support died in the hospital compared with those with two or more sources of support.

Among those who survived and were discharged from the hospital, after six months 53 percent of those with no source of support had died compared with 36 percent of those with one source and 23 percent of those with two or more sources of support. These figures did not change significantly after one year. When the researchers looked at all patients and controlled for other factors that might have influenced survival (such as severity of the heart attack, age, gender, other illnesses, depression, and so on), men and women who reported no emotional support had almost *three times* the mortality risk compared with those who had at least one source of support.[64]

Is this beginning to sound familiar?

Sometimes it is difficult for researchers to separate the effects of lifestyle (diet, exercise, smoking) and social support. In one particularly elegant and definitive study, researchers were able to demonstrate the power of social support independent of other factors.

In the "Ni-Hon-San" study — Nippon (Japan), Honolulu, San Francisco — scientists examined 11,900 Japanese who lived in Nippon and compared them to those who had migrated to Honolulu and to San Francisco. They found that the incidence of heart disease was lowest in Japan, intermediate in Hawaii, and highest in California. At first, it seemed that the closer they came to the American mainland, the sicker they became. This difference was not explained by differences in diet, blood pressure, or cholesterol levels, and they found that the incidence of smoking was actually higher in Japan even though the prevalence of heart disease was lower there.[65]

The researchers then classified the Japanese-Americans in California according to the degree to which they retained a traditional Japanese culture. As in the Roseto study, the most traditional group of Japanese-Americans — in other words, those who maintained their social networks, family ties, and community — had a prevalence of heart disease as low as those living in Japan. In contrast, the group that was most Westernized had a *three-to fivefold increase* in heart disease.[66] In other words, social networks and close family ties protect against disease and premature death.

Thomas Oxman and his colleagues at the University of Texas Medical School examined the relationship of social support and religion to mortality in men and women six months after undergoing elective open-heart surgery (coronary bypass surgery, aortic valve replacement, or both). They asked two questions:

- Do you participate regularly in organized social groups (clubs, church, synagogue, civic activities, and so on)?
- Do you draw strength and comfort from your religious or spiritual faith (whatever religion or spiritual faith that might be)?

They found that those who lacked regular participation in organized social groups had a *fourfold* increased risk of dying six months after surgery, even after controlling for medical factors that might have influenced survival (such as severity of heart disease, age, previous cardiac surgery, and so on). Also, they found that those who did not draw strength and comfort from their religion were *three times* more likely to die six months after surgery.[67]

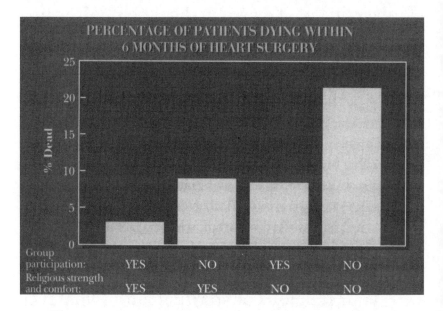

These results indicated that lack of group participation and absence of strength and comfort from religion had independent and additive effects. *Those who neither had regular group participation nor drew strength and comfort from their religion were more than seven times more likely to die six months after surgery.* Seven times! Even though I am unaware of any factor in medicine that causes a sevenfold difference in mortality only six months after open-heart surgery, how many surgeons even ask their patients these two questions in assessing the risk of cardiac surgery?

Love and intimacy can have powerful effects on our health and on our survival even when the interventions are rather modest in intensity or duration. Let's examine a few of these studies.

Lean on Me: Intervention Studies

In 1989, David Spiegel and colleagues at Stanford Medical School published a landmark article in the British journal *The Lancet* in which they studied women with metastatic breast cancer.[68] His intention was to *disprove* the idea that psychosocial interventions could prolong the life of women with breast cancer, in part because Dr. Spiegel was concerned that he was often confused with Dr. Bernie Siegel, who had written several books stating that psychological and social factors could prolong life in cancer patients.[69] Dr. Spiegel wrote, "Our follow-up study was done to investigate whether psychosocial intervention, which significantly reduced anxiety, depression, and pain, would do so without having any effect on the course of the disease."

In this study, women with metastatic breast cancer were randomly assigned to two groups. Both groups received conventional medical care such as chemotherapy, surgery, radiation, and medications. In addition, one group of women met together for ninety minutes once a week for a year. Patients were encouraged to come regularly and to express their feelings about the illness and its effect on their lives in a supportive environment that felt safe enough for them to express what they were really feeling — including their fears of disfigurement, of dying, of being abandoned by their friends and spouse, and so on.

The groups were led by a psychiatrist or social worker plus a therapist who had breast cancer in remission. No one understands what it means to have breast cancer better than others who have gone through similar experiences.

As Dr. Spiegel wrote:

The groups were structured to encourage discussion of how to cope with cancer, but at no time were patients led to believe that participation would affect the course of disease. Group therapy patients were encouraged to come regularly and express their feelings about the illness and the effect on their lives. . . .

Social isolation was countered by developing strong relations among members. . . . Patients focused on how to extract meaning from tragedy by using their experience to help other patients and their families. . . . Clearly, the patients in these groups felt an intense bonding with one another and a sense of acceptance through sharing a common dilemma.

One patient with esophageal strictures (narrowing of the esophagus) due to irradiation described her sense of estrangement from the world; while struggling to swallow soup at a restaurant, she thought, "These people don't realize how fortunate they are just to be able to eat." The therapy group patients visited each other in hospital, wrote poems, and even had a meeting at the home of a dying member. Thus, the groups countered the social isolation that often divides cancer patients from their well-meaning but anxious family and friends.

As a result, a strong sense of community and intimacy developed. Although the "L" word (love) was not used in the journal report, as in most scientific publications, one could say that these women began to love and care for each other.

The groups continued meeting once per

week for just one year. Five years later, Dr. Spiegel told me, "I finally got around to looking at the data, and I almost fell off my chair. Those women who had the weekly support group lived on average *twice as long* as did the other group of women who didn't have the support group."

All of the women in the comparison group (who did not have a support group) were dead after five years; the only women still alive were those who had received the weekly group support sessions. Also, the time interval from first metastasis to death was significantly longer in those who had received the

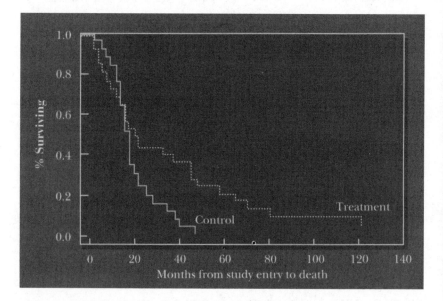

weekly support groups. Dr. Spiegel's work is more fully described in his book, *Living Beyond Limits.*[70]

The investigators also found that a battery of extensive psychological assessments before intervention did not significantly predict survival. The only variable found to affect survival time was participation in the weekly group support sessions.

In a related study, Dr. F. I. Fawzy and colleagues at the UCLA School of Medicine published an article in 1993 evaluating recurrence and survival in patients with malignant melanoma who had participated in a

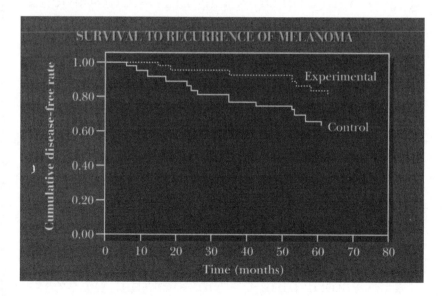

six-week group intervention five to six years earlier.[71] Patients whose malignant melanoma had been surgically removed were randomly assigned to a support group or to a comparison group. None of the patients in either group received any kind of conventional treatment other than surgery.

As in Dr. Spiegel's study, patients in the support group met for ninety minutes weekly, but only for six weeks rather than one year. Five to six years later, those who had participated in the six-week group support sessions had a statistically significantly better survival rate than the comparison group. Only three of the thirty-four patients who had received the six-week support group had died after five to six years, compared with ten of the patients in the comparison group — more than *three times* as many. Also, although not statistically significant due to the relatively small sample size, a definite trend in the same direction was noted for recurrence: seven of the patients who had received the support group experienced recurrence compared with thirteen of the comparison group — almost twice as many.

It is astonishing to consider that six weeks of group support could have a major effect on prolonging survival and preventing recurrence five to six years later in patients with

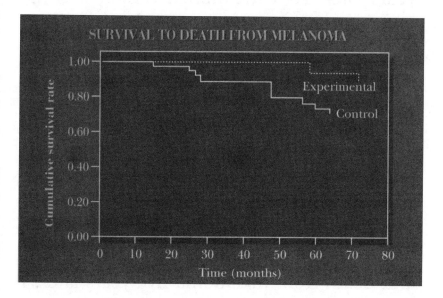

SURVIVAL TO DEATH FROM MELANOMA

malignant melanoma — or that one year of group support could double the length of survival in women with metastatic breast cancer five years later — yet that is what these carefully controlled studies have shown.

In a way, the Spiegel and Fawzy studies are the counterpart of the studies of Harvard and Johns Hopkins students that I described earlier. Just as the studies of the warmth and closeness of these students' relationships with their parents affected the frequency of diseases thirty-five to fifty years later, the Fawzy and Spiegel studies demonstrate that even a few weeks of social support can affect recurrence and survival from cancer many years later. As I mentioned earlier, it is the ongoing pattern of how we relate to others and to ourselves that is such a powerful determinant of health and illness — even life and death. Most people relate to others now pretty much the same as they did earlier in life. We do not get much training in school or other places in how to be loving and intimate in our relationships. If we don't change something, it's likely to continue.

However, even six weeks of training in the Fawzy study had an impact on recurrence and death from melanoma five years later. I don't believe that the six-week intervention itself was so powerful. During the six weeks of intervention, the melanoma patients learned how to communicate more effectively and — equally important — how good it feels to be in a nurturing, loving, intimate environment where they could feel safe enough to let down their emotional defenses in order to give and receive love more freely and more fully. This awareness motivated them to begin incorporating these skills and values into their daily lives even after the six weeks were completed. As I will describe in chapter 4, there are many ways of changing these lifelong patterns, including group support, psychological support, communication skills, selfless service, and other methods.

Both studies considered other possible explanations for what they observed. Dr. Spiegel found no significant differences when controlling for staging (severity) at time of entry, chemotherapy, radiation, or other factors. Dr. Fawzy acknowledged that the intervention could have fostered improved health habits such as avoiding the sun, better nutrition, increased exercise, or stress management, but there was no evidence that any of these occurred.

As I mentioned in chapter 1, if a pharmaceutical company found that drug X doubled the length of survival in women with metastatic breast cancer, almost every doctor would be prescribing it. Further, imagine that patients took drug X for only six weeks, yet five to six years later it prolonged survival in malignant melanoma. Full-page ads would proclaim the benefits in medical journals and news magazines. Yet, despite Dr. Spiegel's important efforts in training other health professionals, most medical schools do not teach students the importance of love and intimacy.

As one group of researchers wrote recently:

It is clear that group psychological therapies improve the quality of life of many participating cancer patients, and there is preliminary evidence that it may prolong life in some cases. Support groups, while becoming more common, have generally been an "extra," not an integral part of cancer management, and not strongly advocated; as a result, only a very small proportion of patients attend them. However, with the increasing evidence for benefits of psychological therapy, and the lack of harmful side-effects, it can be argued that this kind of help might reasonably be advocated and provided for all patients who will accept it. We propose that it is time to consider psychological therapy as an adjuvant in cancer management, analogous to adjuvant chemotherapy.[72]

Group support may be particularly beneficial in cancer patients. People who have been recently diagnosed with cancer may find it hard to get emotional support when they most need it. When someone is diagnosed with cancer, he or she often feels stigmatized. One patient told me, "I feel like I've left the community of the well and I've gone into the desert of the diseased" because many of those she thought were her friends began to withdraw or react inappropriately when they learned of her breast cancer.

In another important study, more than two thousand middle-aged men employed at the Western Electric Company in Chicago were given a questionnaire in the 1950s to assess a number of psychological and emotional factors, including depression.

Twenty years later, those who were found to have been emotionally depressed at the baseline examination were twice as likely to have died from cancer of all types during the twenty years of follow-up.[73] Several studies have demonstrated that people with cancer have a higher incidence of depression, but this is not surprising since the diagnosis of cancer itself is often depressing. One of the important design features of this study was that people did not have cancer at the time they were undergoing psychological testing. Their depression *preceded* the development of cancer and, thus, may have been a factor in causing it.

This association did not vary appreciably in magnitude among the early (1958–1962), middle (1963–1968), and later (1969–1974) years of follow-up. Also, it persisted after adjustment for age, cigarette smoking, use of alcohol, family history of cancer, and occupational status, and it was not specific to any particular site or type of cancer.[74] Of interest is that these scientists found that psychological *repression* was not associated with an increased risk of cancer even though psychological *depression* clearly was.

In a related study, more than two hundred women with breast cancer diagnosed between 1958 and 1960 were interviewed at that time about the amount of stress and social support they had in the five years preceding their diagnosis. The researchers found that social involvement and social support were independently related to survival twenty years later.[75]

Another psychological factor that had a profound influence on premature death and disease was hostility. Those who scored in the upper twenty percent of hostility when tested twenty years earlier had a forty-two percent increased risk of premature death *from all causes combined*, including heart disease and cancer, when compared to those who scored in the lower twenty percent of hostility. These relationships persisted even after adjusting for other factors that might have influenced mortality, including age, blood pressure, serum cholesterol level, cigarette smoking, and intake of alcohol.

In an analysis of over forty-five studies,

hostility has emerged as one of the most important personality variables in coronary heart disease.[76] The effects of hostility are equal to or greater in magnitude to the traditional risk factors for heart disease: elevated cholesterol levels, high blood pressure, and so on.[77]

I believe that hostility is a manifestation of a more fundamental issue: loneliness and isolation. People who feel lonely and isolated are often angry and hostile; when they act with chronic anger and hostility, it tends to drive people away, causing them to feel even more lonely and isolated in a vicious cycle.[78]

Dealing with the underlying loneliness can be healing. A review of several programs that reduced cardiac deaths by fifty percent or more after a heart attack found that regardless of their approach, all such programs shared a common therapeutic mechanism: providing emotional support during a period of high vulnerability to stress.[79]

Another review of nine published studies found a dose-response relationship between the extent of social networks and the risk of cardiovascular disease — the more well-developed the social ties, the less heart disease.[80] Other researchers found something similar: "Risk varies in a graded fashion as a function of the social contacts score and is independent of a number of risk factors [such as cholesterol, blood pressure, etc.] and other potential confounders."[81]

One such program was the Recurrent Coronary Prevention Project (RCCP), directed by Meyer Friedman, M.D., who pioneered the concept of what he termed "type A behavior." This behavior pattern included a sense of time urgency, talking fast, doing several things at the same time, not liking to stand in line, and other related behaviors. At first, type A behavior was thought to be a risk factor for heart disease. Later research demonstrated that one component of type A behavior — hostility — accounted for most of the increased risk. (This was good news for nonhostile type A's like me.)

In 1978, Dr. Friedman and his colleagues began a four-and-a-half year study to determine if men who had suffered a heart attack could reduce the likelihood of another and thus increase their survival by changing type A behavior. Patients were divided into three groups: One group received only advice and information concerning diet, exercise, drugs, possible surgical regimens, and cardiovascular pathophysiology. A second group received the same and also participated in support groups that provided advice on changing type A behavior and techniques for enhancing self-esteem. A third group received nothing.

What did they find? After four and one-half years, patients who received only advice and information had a 21.2 percent recurrence rate of heart attacks and those who received nothing had a 28.2 percent recurrence rate. However, those who had attended the support group had only a 12.9 percent recurrence rate — 54 percent less than the group that received nothing.[82]

While it is impossible to separate how much of this effect was from modifying type A behavior and how much from the love and emotional support received by this group, some insight can be gained by how two of the principal investigators described the most important characteristic of a group leader: "Perhaps more than any other thing a leader can do for these patients is to provide them with what many did not adequately secure in childhood — unconditional love and affection from a respected parent figure."[83, 84]

Dr. Friedman described the field director in this way:

Diane Ulmer became a sort of surrogate mother to hundreds of our male participants. While we had been aware of the importance of inadequate maternal love and affection in the formation of type A behavior in men, we did not realize until we were well along in the study that such deprivation could be to some degree compensated for in adult life. . . . However, the wives of our male participants were rarely able to fill the role, one reason being that many of them were themselves type A, and thus busy searching for (and not finding) the unconditional parental love missing in their own childhoods.[85]

In addition to hostility, researchers have found that cynicism and suspiciousness are the other toxic components of type A behavior. In one study, for example, five hundred men and women were followed for fifteen years. Those individuals with scores indicating higher levels of suspiciousness had greater mortality risk. This association remained significant after controlling for age, sex, physician's ratings of functional health, smoking, cholesterol, and alcohol intake. In addition, suspiciousness was associated with physician's ratings of health at the initiation of follow-up.[86]

Why? As I described earlier, we can be intimate only to the degree that we can be open and vulnerable. It can be frightening to make yourself vulnerable to someone, for when you feel vulnerable you might get hurt.

When you make a commitment to some-one, you feel safer and more trusting. You are more likely to risk being vulnerable and open to the love that longs to flow from your heart to your beloved's and back again — and the resulting intimacy can be healing. On the other hand, when you feel mistrusting and cynical, it's hard to remain open and vulnerable. The resulting isolation can lead to illness and premature death. In short:

---

commitment → trust → vulnerability →
   intimacy → healing;

fear / no commitment →
   mistrust / cynicism → hostility →
   closed off → isolation →
   disease / premature death

Infectious Love

Social ties — that is, love and intimacy — with friends, family, work, and community may help protect against infectious diseases as well. To test this idea, Dr. Sheldon Cohen and his colleagues at Carnegie-Mellon University and the University of Pittsburgh recruited 276 healthy volunteers ranging in age from eighteen to fifty-five. The volunteers were given nasal drops containing rhinovirus — the virus that causes the common cold. (Subjects were paid to be part of this experiment.)

The investigators assessed participation in twelve types of social relationships. These included relationships with a spouse, parents, parents-in-law, children, other close family members, close neighbors, friends, workmates, schoolmates, fellow volunteers in charity or community work, members of groups without religious affiliations (social, recreational, or professional), and members of religious groups. One point was given for each type of relationship when a person spoke (in person or by phone) to someone in that category at least once every two weeks, so the maximum score was twelve points. Also, the total number of people with whom they spoke at least once every two weeks was counted.

Almost all of the people who were exposed to the rhinovirus were infected by it, but not everyone who was infected developed the signs and symptoms of a cold. The number of social relationships played a powerful role in protecting people who were infected from developing a cold.

Those reporting only one to three types of relationships had more than *four times* the risk of developing a cold than those reporting six or more types of relationships. Those having four to five types of relationships had an intermediate risk of developing a cold. These differences were not fully explained by antibody titers, smoking, exercise, amount of sleep, alcohol, vitamin C, or other factors.

The diversity of relationships (having multiple types of relationships) was more important than the total number of people with whom they spoke at least once every two weeks. In short, social support increased their resistance to developing a cold even when they were infected with a virus that causes it.[87]

Why? Dr. Janice Kiecolt-Glaser and Dr. Ronald Glaser have conducted some of the most interesting studies documenting the effects of relationships on the immune system. In one study, for example, they found that couples who had been married for an average of forty-two years and constantly argued had weakened immune systems. "You might expect that arguments would have less impact on older couples because they've gone through these disagreements many times before and have learned to deal with them," they wrote, "but that's not the case."[88]

On the other end of the marriage spectrum, they studied ninety newlywed couples who were admitted to a hospital research unit for twenty-four hours. (I don't know about you, but I wouldn't want to spend my honeymoon in a research unit. . . .) Those who exhibited more negative or hostile behaviors during a thirty-minute discussion of marital problems showed greater decreases over twenty-four hours on four functional immunological assays.

In other words, your immune system is less effective when you are in conflict with your spouse or companion, even when you just got married and you are otherwise happy. Instead of being a source of refuge, love, and support, it is particularly distressing when your spouse is a source of conflict. Women were more likely to show negative immunological changes than men. Also, the most negative couples had larger increases in blood pressure that remained elevated longer.[89]

Dr. David McClelland and his colleagues conducted a fascinating series of studies showing the power of relationships to affect immunity. They asked students to watch a documentary movie about Mother Teresa's service to the sick and dying poor of Calcutta's worst slums. Another group of students watched a more neutral film. On average, those who watched the movie about Mother Teresa showed a significant increase in protective antibodies whereas those who watched the neutral film did not.[90]

However, not all students who saw the film about Mother Teresa showed improvement in immune function. Some actually got worse. The researchers wondered why.

After students watched the Mother Teresa documentary, the researchers then showed the students a photograph of a couple sitting on a bench by a river and asked them to write a story about this couple to gain greater insight into each student's unconscious perceptions and projections.

What did they find? Those who wrote stories depicting the couple in a happy, trusting relationship who helped each other, respected each other, and shared warm, loving feelings had the biggest increases in immune antibodies. They also reported fewer infectious diseases during the preceding year. Those who wrote stories in which the couple manipulated, deceived, and abandoned each other showed the biggest decreases in antibodies and reported significantly more illness during the previous year.[91, 92] How they perceived the couple in this photograph was a good barometer of how they perceived the world in general.

Once again, this study demonstrated the power of our perceptions — how we view ourselves in relation to others. Two people watching the same movie or looking at the same photograph — or, for that matter, existing in the same job, family, or city — may have completely different life experiences based on their level of mistrust and suspicion.

In short, believing that the world is a dangerous place helps to make it so in a self-fulfilling prophecy. How we perceive relationships can affect our health and our survival.

Labor of Love

Several studies have shown that social support can improve the outcome of pregnancy and childbirth. In a review of over 144 studies, Drs. Hoffman and Hatch at Columbia University concluded that intimate social support from a partner or family member substantially improves fetal growth. In contrast, stressful life events during pregnancy do not increase the risk of premature birth when women feel loved and supported.[93]

One of the first studies was conducted in 1972 on 170 U.S. Army wives at a military hospital. They were given a questionnaire before their sixth month of pregnancy to assess how much emotional and psychological support they had. The women who reported many life changes in the years preceding pregnancy and who did not report much emotional and psychological support had *three times* as many complications of childbirth as those who had more support.[94]

At the University of Arizona, researchers studied teenage Navajo mothers who were pregnant and unmarried. After giving birth, the mothers who had low to medium levels of social support had *four times* the number of complications as the mothers who had high levels of social support.[95, 96]

In Guatemala City, two studies revealed that the continuous presence of a supportive companion during labor and delivery shortened the duration of labor and reduced the need for cesarean section and other interventions. In Guatemala City, it was routine for women to undergo labor alone, without family, friends, spouse, or even nurse support, so this provided researchers with an opportunity to find out the effects of a supportive companion during labor and delivery. In one study, forty women were randomly divided into two groups. One group was left alone; women in the other group received constant emotional support from admission to delivery by a friendly companion the woman had not previously met (known as a "doula"). The duration of labor in the group of women left alone was 19.3 hours, compared with only 8.7 hours for the women with the doula. Also, the mothers with the doula were more likely to smile, stroke, and talk to their infant children than those in the other group.[97, 98]

This approach was replicated and studied in greater depth at the Cleveland Clinic. Approximately four hundred healthy pregnant women in labor were randomly assigned either to a group that received the continuous support of a doula or to a group that was monitored by an inconspicuous observer — in other words, they were given similar medical attention but without the emotional support. Another two hundred women were assigned to a comparison group who received neither emotional support nor close monitoring.

Only eight percent of those in the continuous emotional support group had cesarean sections compared with thirteen percent of the observed group and eighteen percent of the comparison group. Even more striking, only eight percent of those in the continuous emotional support group needed epidural anesthesia compared with twenty-three percent of the observed group and fifty-five percent of the comparison group. Duration of labor, prolonged infant hospitalization, induced labor, and maternal fever followed a similar pattern — a threefold to sixfold difference.[99]

Would your insurance company pay for a doula to give you continuous emotional support during pregnancy? Would a 300–600 percent reduction in complications of childbirth have cost the insurance company less than the cost of a doula? Did your doctor or nurse encourage you to bring a friend, spouse, or other family to the hospital?

I learned how to deliver babies at a county hospital. It was "watch one, do one, teach one." I delivered fifty-three babies in four weeks at the beginning of my third year of medical school. The women were lined up in a row of gurneys, one after another. Not a companion to be found. At that time, a mother was separated from her husband and other family members during labor and delivery. During the past twenty years, many hospitals have set up birthing centers that encourage family members to become more involved in the process of childbirth in response to the demands of people who wanted a more caring and compassionate experience.

In a more detailed study, Nancy Collins and her colleagues at UCLA conducted a prospective study of 129 ethnically diverse, economically disadvantaged pregnant women to see if social support would improve physical and mental outcomes in pregnancy. They found that women who received more prenatal social support and those who were more satisfied with that support experienced fewer difficulties in labor, delivered babies of higher birth weight, and gave birth to healthier babies as indicated by their Apgar rating. Also, those who received more social support during pregnancy reported less depression after childbirth.[100]

The *amount* of support that mothers received was important, but even more significant was the mothers' satisfaction with the *quality* of that support. Those who were more satisfied with that support delivered babies with higher Apgar scores. Women who were dissatisfied with the prenatal support they received, especially from the baby's father, were more likely to have experienced postpartum depression. As found in other studies described earlier in this chapter, the mother's *perception* of how much emotional support she had was more important than objective measures of it in determining the incidence of premature births and birth complications.

Several other studies have found that social support during pregnancy improves the growth of the fetus.[101, 102] One study, for example, found that the likelihood of fetal growth retardation was almost *five times greater* in the absence of partner support.[103] Other studies documented that social support can affect the duration of pregnancy. In a London study, rates of preterm delivery were significantly lower among women with a partner-confidant than among those without, and increased contact with neighbors was also protective.[104] Another study showed that both partner support and being married significantly increased the duration of pregnancy.[105]

Petter or Pettee?

The beneficial effects of social support, love, and intimacy are not limited to humans. A number of studies demonstrated that people who have pets are healthier than those who do not.

The Cardiac Arrhythmia Suppression Trial (CAST) studied men and women who had sustained a heart attack and who had irregular heartbeats. Only one of the eighty-seven people (1.1 percent) who owned dogs died during the study compared with nineteen of the 282 people (6.7 percent) who did not own dogs — over *six times* as many![106] This study also found that the amount of social support from humans also was an independent predictor of survival in these patients.

Ironically, the drugs that were tested — encainide and flecainide — actually caused an *increase* in cardiac deaths and the study had to be stopped prematurely. If these drugs had shown a sixfold decrease in deaths, you can be pretty sure that just about every doctor in the country would be prescribing them for patients with heart attacks and irregular heartbeats. Yet when was the last time that your doctor prescribed a pet or a supportive friend for you?

An earlier study focused on patients who were recently hospitalized with a heart attack or chest pain. After one year, only 6 percent of the pet owners died compared with 28 percent of the patients who did not own pets — over *four times* as many people who did not own pets were dead compared with those who had one. This finding was independent of disease severity, exercise, or other known factors.[107]

Pet owners who received Medicaid benefits made fewer visits to their physicians than nonowners.[108] Having a pet causes decreased cardiovascular reactivity (such as blood pressure response).[109] In one study, the effect of a dog on lowering blood pressure reactivity was even greater than the presence of a good friend — since the friend was often perceived as judgmental whereas the dog was not.[110]

For many people, their pet may be as close as they get to what these researchers in their most clinical jargon termed "nonevaluative social support" — in other words, the experience of unconditional, nonjudgmental love.

Just as humans respond beneficially to the love of animals, so do animals to humans. In 1980, *Science*, one of the most well-respected and prestigious journals, published a fascinating article revealing the effects of social factors on the progression of atherosclerosis (blockages in the arteries).

In this study, the scientists put a group of rabbits on a diet rich in cholesterol. The rabbits were genetically comparable, so the scientists expected all of them to get blocked arteries at about the same rate — but they didn't. Some of the rabbits got a lot more blockages than others, and the scientists couldn't figure out why since they were all on the same diet and they all had similar genes.

The rabbits were stacked in cages up to the ceiling. The ones in the higher cages got a lot more blockages than the ones in the lower cages. At first, that made no sense to them. When they looked into it further, they found that when the lab technician — who was short — was feeding the rabbits, she would play with the ones in the lower cages because she could reach them but ignore the ones higher up. They thought, Well, maybe that had something to do with it.

So they took another group of rabbits and randomly divided them into three groups (A, B, and C) and then repeated the experiment later with two groups (D and E). All of the rabbits were put on the same high-cholesterol diet. As before, they were genetically comparable. Rabbits in groups C and E were left alone other than for normal laboratory care. The rabbits in groups A, B, and D were taken out of their cages every day. Here's what the experimenters wrote:

It should be noted that the essence of the experimental environment studied here was to establish a one-to-one relationship between each animal and the experimenter. This was achieved through an early morning, half-hour visit during which each animal was handled, stroked, talked to, and played with; an hour-long feeding period during which the animal was also touched and talked to; and a number of five-minute visits during the day. Through this daily process, the animals quickly learned to recognize the experimenter, and when she was present, many even sought her personal attention.

In other words, the researcher touched them, talked to them, petted them, played with them, caressed them, loved them — and then killed them to look at their arteries. (One reason why I don't do animal experiments . . .) The researchers were amazed to find that these rabbits had 60 percent less plaque in their arteries than those that were ignored, even though they were genetically comparable and on the same diet. Also, blood pressure, serum cholesterol levels, and heart rate were comparable in both groups, so the effects of the love and support were not mediated through these physiological mechanisms.[111] Something else was going on. So, whether you are the petter or the pettee, you are less likely to need a PET scan. . . .

In a more brutal set of experiments, researchers in Houston demonstrated how social support can help protect against even extremes of danger and disease. The researchers induced heart attacks in pigs. Afterwards, those pigs that were in a laboratory with staff who were familiar to them did not develop lethal irregular heartbeats, whereas pigs who were moved to a new laboratory with unfamiliar lab workers often died from fatal irregular heartbeats.[112] Thus, social support can increase survival in pigs even after inflicted with heart attacks.

Touch is important to humans as well. The simple act of touching someone is a powerful way to begin healing loneliness and isolation. While the most important benefits of touching may be beyond measurement, some can be observed and studied.

The experience of being in an intensive care unit is a powerfully isolating one for many people because they spend much of their time alone. When a doctor or nurse or technician appears, the tubes and wires and machinery often become the focus of most of their time and attention.

In a series of studies in intensive care units, Dr. James Lynch and his colleagues studied men and women who had significant irregular heartbeats called ventricular arrhythmias and were under constant monitoring in the coronary care unit. They found that a significant reduction in irregular heartbeats occurred when the nurse or doctor touched the patients to take their pulse. In some of these patients, pulse taking had the power to completely suppress irregular heartbeats that had previously been occurring.[113] Dr. Lynch's book, *The Broken Heart,* is a wonderful exposition of the fact that "reflected in our hearts there is a biological basis for our need to form loving human relationships. If we fail to fulfill that need, our health is in peril."[114]

In summary, love promotes survival. Both nurturing and being nurtured are life-affirming. Anything that takes you outside of yourself promotes healing — in profound ways that can be measured — independent of other known factors such as diet and exercise.

There are many more studies I could cite. Indeed, several books have been written summarizing the scientific and medical literature on the health-damaging consequences of loneliness and isolation and the life-enhancing power of love and intimacy in whatever technical terms these concepts are expressed.[115–120]

I only want to include enough studies to make it clear that there is a strong scientific basis documenting that these ideas matter — across all ages from infants to the most elderly, in all parts of the world, in all strata of life. The rest of this book explores why love and intimacy play such a powerful role in our lives and how we can find ways of healing what separates us from ourselves, from each other, and from our true Self.

In the next chapter, I describe part of my own personal journey in learning to open my heart. Why was I so afraid of what I most wanted?

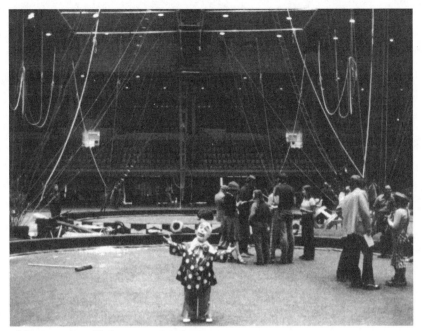

Clown Auditions, 1975

3

"It's You!"

What good is it for a man to gain the whole world, yet forfeit his soul?
— MARK 8:36

There are many paths to wisdom, but each begins with a broken heart.
— LEONARD COHEN

In the middle of life's way, I found myself in a dark woods where the right way was lost.

— DANTE, *Inferno*

I have loved, and I have been loved, and all the rest is just background music.

— ESTELLE RAMEY

On my fortieth birthday, I thought my dreams were coming true. During that week:

My third book reached number one on the *New York Times* best-seller list.

My colleagues and I received a letter from the American Heart Association informing us that they accepted our latest research findings for their annual scientific meeting: We had found even more reversal of heart disease in our research patients after four years than after one year. They planned a press conference to announce our results.

I was invited to spend the night at the White House.

Two weeks before, our research had been featured on the front page of the *New York Times* and on all of the evening news shows when Mutual of Omaha announced they would cover our program for reversing heart disease, the first time a major insurance company paid for an alternative medicine treatment. Later, *USA Today* ran a front-page headline, "PATIENT CALLS ORNISH PROGRAM 'MIRACULOUS.'"

I went to my twenty-fifth anniversary high school reunion. The former captain of the football team — who wouldn't give me the time of day when we were in high school together — came up to me, gave me a big hug, and boomed, "Gee, Dean, I should have been nicer to you in high school but I didn't know you were going to be so successful!"

So . . . why was I feeling so lonely, unsatisfied, and discontented?

Unhappiness was no stranger to me. When I was nineteen, I became profoundly depressed and almost committed suicide. I wrote about this time in my life in chapter 5 of an earlier book, *Dr. Dean Ornish's Program for Reversing Heart Disease*, which was published in 1990. It was a little scary to be that self-disclosing. After all, like most people, I usually want to show my best side, not my darkest moments.

Since the publication of that book, I have received thousands of letters from people, many of whom wrote to say that this particular chapter was the most meaningful and useful for them. Having a greater understanding of the process I went through often gave them more insight into their own lives. Also, my willingness to be self-revealing made it easier for them to be.

To me, the story of someone's journey of growth and discovery is usually more interesting than hearing them give a sermon on the mount. I want to know *how* he learned — the experiences he had, the mistakes he made — not just what he now knows.

In that spirit, I want to share with you the process of what I have been learning in more recent years. Part of me hesitates to do so because I do not want to seem either self-aggrandizing or foolish, although there are times when I am each of these. Nevertheless, I decided to write this chapter in hopes that this phase of my journey may be of some value to you. Of course, this is still an on-going process. Perhaps these experiences may help you avoid some of my mistakes. (You can make new ones!)

One of the most painful aspects of being nineteen was feeling stupid, like a fraud. Somehow, I believed, I had managed to fool people into thinking that I was smart when I was really an imposter. Now that I was at a university with what seemed like *really smart* people, where over half the student body graduated first or second in their high school classes, it was only a matter of time before they figured out what a mistake they had made in admitting me. I felt unworthy and ashamed of my unworthiness.

Even more terrifying than the feelings of inadequacy was a deeper level of suffering: a crisis of the spirit. I had a clear vision at age nineteen that *no accomplishments or material rewards would ever bring me lasting peace and happiness.* This spiritual realization is at the heart of virtually all religious and spiritual traditions, yet it was too much for me to handle at such a young age.

It was bad enough to believe that I would never amount to anything. Worse was realizing that it wouldn't matter anyway. This double whammy caused me to become profoundly depressed at age nineteen.

In some ways, it would have been more consoling to believe that some things *would* make me happy even if I thought I never could attain them than to understand that they wouldn't bring lasting happiness even if I did. I realized that even if I got everything our culture says will bring joy — name, fame, accomplishments, sex, power, money — the pleasure wouldn't last.

For a brief moment, it really does seem like getting these things brings happiness and removes pain, which reinforces that belief. It *is* fun for a short while, which is what makes it so seductive. By analogy, taking nitroglycerin relieves chest pain temporarily and makes you think that your health comes from the medication. Aspirin temporarily relieves the headache.

Unfortunately, the happiness and well-being are usually fleeting. They do not last, at least not for long. Fifteen minutes, maybe a few weeks — soon followed by, "Now what?" It's never enough. Or: "So what?" Why bother? Who cares? Big deal. Nothing matters. I was left with nihilism and despair.

One of the most frightening aspects of being this depressed is that you really believe that you're seeing the world clearly for the first time. Life is awful, and it is *always* going to be that way. Suffering. Death. Disease. War. Violence. Poverty. Horror. That's all I could see at that time.

This distortion of reality is what leads to the feelings of helplessness and hopelessness that are the hallmark of severe depression. I was convinced that every time I had thought I was happy or might ever be happy was delusional; I had just been fooling myself. All the times I thought I might find meaning or purpose had been misguided.

From Breakdown to Breakthrough

This suffering became a doorway for me to begin transforming my life and to take my first steps on a spiritual path. In January 1972, I was so depressed that I withdrew from college and went to my parents' home to recuperate. I will always remain grateful to them for taking me in at a time when I most needed it.

My older sister had benefited greatly from studying yoga and meditation with Sri Swami Satchidananda, an eminent and ecumenical spiritual teacher, so my parents held a reception in his honor at their home. There is an old saying, "When the student is ready, the teacher appears," and that was clearly true for me.

He gave a short lecture in their living room and began by saying, "Nothing can bring you lasting peace." It felt validating to hear that, but I was profoundly depressed and he seemed radiantly happy. He went on to say the other half of the equation: *"Nothing can bring lasting peace, but you have it already if you just stop disturbing it. It is there always."* That moment changed my life. I decided to study with him. I had nothing to lose; I figured I could always kill myself if he were wrong.

A few months later, I began studying yoga and meditation with him, and he also advised me to begin a vegetarian diet. I didn't know at the time that I was beginning a spiritual journey; I only wanted to make the emotional pain go away, so I was ready to try just about anything. I learned that with the right guidance and support, a breakdown can become a breakthrough.

At first, I had a hard time sitting still long enough even to practice yoga and meditation. One of the great paradoxes is that, being unaware of the source of my well-being, I was disturbing the peace that was already there by running after so many things I had been told would bring it to me. On a practical level, the anxiety, fear, and worry that resulted from disturbing my peace made it more difficult to get the things I was running after, or to enjoy them very much when they came.

Over time, though, I began to get glimpses of what it meant to feel moments of inner peace. I realized that those moments of calm weren't something I got from outside myself; rather, I temporarily quieted down my mind and body enough during meditation to stop disturbing what is already there, always.

Discovering this truth was one thing. Understanding it and integrating it into my life was another.

Although I had experienced at age nineteen that nothing material from the outside would bring lasting happiness, it was an overwhelming realization, so I pretended to myself that it wasn't true. I didn't want to believe it. Deep down, I began to doubt my own vision of this truth.

I wondered: maybe getting and doing enough *would* bring happiness. Maybe people just told themselves that these things wouldn't bring happiness in order to make themselves feel better for not getting and doing all that — sour grapes. And even if it wasn't *lasting* happiness, maybe enough moments of temporary happiness could be strung together to fill up much of a lifetime.

A few months later, I went back to college. Meditation and yoga helped me stay so much more calm and focused that I was able to graduate *summa cum laude* and gave the commencement address. During the next twenty years, I had many accomplishments.

Yet I was no freer than when I was profoundly depressed in college and thought I would never amount to anything. I was in a golden cage rather than a steel one, but a cage nonetheless. I was still looking in the wrong places for happiness and peace, even though I knew better. To paraphrase the

Indian sage Ramana Maharshi earlier in this century, looking to external attainments to provide lasting happiness without discovering one's true Self is like trying to cover the whole world with leather to avoid the pain of walking on stones and thorns. It is much simpler to wear shoes.

The loneliness could not be fed for long by external accomplishments and activities, no matter how interesting or exciting. Not that I didn't try. I worked at least eighty hours a week, sometimes more, which was a good distraction from these feelings. I remember rushing to catch a plane and just making it inside as the door was being closed.

"You look harried," the flight attendant told me.

"I *feel* harried," I replied.

"Well," she said, not recognizing me, "I just read this book by Dr. Dean Ornish. I highly recommend it. It has some wonderful stress management techniques in there that might be helpful for you."

"Yes, I'm familiar with that book. . . ."

God's little reminder.

The irony was not lost on me. Although I was quite healthy, I was increasingly stressed. I began to imagine the headlines: "AUTHOR OF *STRESS, DIET, & YOUR*

HEART GETS HEART ATTACK FROM STRESS DESPITE EXCELLENT DIET."

I came to the end of the myth on my fortieth birthday. The contrast between what I was achieving and what I was feeling was so great that I could no longer pretend to myself that these things would bring happiness. I could no longer continue as I had been. I couldn't tell myself, "Gee, maybe if I accomplished more, *then* I'd be happy." I had succeeded way beyond my earlier dreams.

The extremes of worldly success and inner turmoil were impossible to ignore — as if the universe were saying, "Hey, Dean — listen up! Pay attention! Can I make it any clearer for you?"

Why was I so dissatisfied? Could that wise inner voice that had spoken to me at age nineteen have been right? All those accomplishments, all that stuff, all the fame and fortune that were supposed to bring happiness did not bring lasting meaning, lasting joy, lasting peace.

I had moments of satisfaction and joy, of course, but not with any continuity. It was very gratifying and meaningful to know that the research and the books and the other work my colleagues and I were doing were remarkably beneficial to so many people. We were able to help them live happier lives, rediscover inner sources of peace and joy, and often begin healing their physical, emotional, and spiritual pain — but not my own. I was missing what was the most meaningful. I didn't have the depth of love and intimacy I desired in the relationship that was most important to me. I was afraid to open my heart.

Physician, Heal Thyself

The disconnect between how much I was able to help others and how little I was able to help myself in this area became a catalyst and a crucible for the next phase in my journey.

Over time, years of meditation gave me glimpses of the interconnectedness and interdependence of all life. I experienced that on one level we are alone, separate, *apart from* everyone and everything; on another level, we are the Self in different disguises, different names and forms, *a part of* everyone and everything. Many religions proclaim as a fundamental truth, "The Lord is One."

This experience of interconnectedness is part of spiritual traditions and the perennial wisdom in virtually all religions and cultures. Albert Einstein wrote,

A human being is a part of the whole that we call the universe, a part limited in time and space. He experiences himself, his thoughts and feelings, as something separated from the rest — a kind of optical illusion of his consciousness. This illusion is a prison for us, restricting us to our personal desires and to affection for only the few people nearest us. Our task must be to free ourselves from this prison by widening our circle of compassion to embrace all living beings and all of nature.

Although these glimpses of transcendent experiences meant a lot to me and gave me hope and awareness, they did not last. I could feel the peace of experiencing this oneness, but, like a visitor in someone else's home, I couldn't stay there for very long. I know now that I first needed to learn how to more fully be human. Trying to skip that stage was like trying to pretend I was not feeling angry and going straight to forgiveness without first allowing myself to be human and to acknowledge the feelings. I needed to get out of my head and into my heart.

A friend of mine who struggles with similar issues sent me the following as part of a letter:

My way is always to retreat into my head. Into a cold space that thinks instead of feels. I imagine you do the same thing. This is an incredibly hard thing for others to be around, particularly when those of us behaving this way are people who have a warm exterior and presence, then become cooler closer in. I often feel safety retreating into work . . . something I know and like doing, something I can succeed at by pouring life energies in.

But the mind is ultimately a less satisfying place than the heart. And the mind can often have anger at the bottom, while the heart, at the bottom, has compassion. There were times on my trip that I felt like a volcano — molten lava ready to erupt.

From Passion to Compassion

I dated a lot in high school and college, like many people in my generation. At first, it seemed liberating to go out with different people. After a while, though, I began to realize that what I thought was bringing me the most freedom was exactly what was most limiting and binding me. I later learned that what seemed to be the most confining —

commitment, discipline, and monogamy —
were actually the most liberating and joyful.
In high school and college, though, these
words sounded dry, boring, confining, and
limiting. I wanted to feel free and *enjoy* life.

In my generation, many people asked,
"Why have any self-imposed limitations
when you don't have to? Why not eat anything and everything you want? Why not do
everything you want to do?"

I am learning that we had it backwards.
Consciously *choosing* commitment, discipline, and monogamy can be liberating.
There is great freedom in these words. Why?
Freely choosing discipline gives more power
— power to create, to express, to enjoy. A
musician who spends hours practicing can
express himself or herself in new ways that
nourish the soul. Freely choosing commitment and monogamy creates safety and
makes intimacy possible.

Intimacy is liberating and healing, but only
if you feel safe. "Opening your heart" is just
another way of saying that you are willing to
let down your emotional defenses and allow
yourself to be emotionally vulnerable. As I
described in the previous chapter, you can
only be intimate to the degree that you can
be vulnerable. You can be vulnerable and
open your heart only to the degree that you

feel safe — because if you make yourself vulnerable, you might get hurt.

I was having a superficial experience in high school and college by going out with different women. Going out with more than one woman helped buffer intimacy. If I got too close to one person and thus became too vulnerable, then I could go back to another one. Push-pull. I was neither alone nor too intimate. It was usually fun in the moment but often left me feeling even more empty and lonely.

Like a medication that provides temporary relief but soon creates its own need, I found myself caught in a vicious cycle. The temporary relief from emotional pain and loneliness that an evening out, an award, or an accomplishment could provide was what made these so seductive. How do *you* spell relief?

In a strange way, I found it easier to be open and intimate with someone I didn't know very well than being in a long-term relationship. I didn't have a history with a new person; we hadn't spent years hurting each other and closing down parts of ourselves to protect those soft spots. But the intimacy was limited and without continuity.

Why was I so afraid of the intimacy that I most desired?

Like many people, I grew up in a loving family without many personal or emotional boundaries — what I affectionately call "The Ornish Blob." In every family there is a process of how each person individuates and separates from the rest of the family. This was my form of the task, which was not unique to me.

In one sense, the lack of personal boundaries felt warm, fuzzy, comfortable, like living inside a big bowl of warm oatmeal. In another, though, it went beyond that. As in many families, I began to realize that I did not have a very well-formed sense of having a separate self. Over time, I learned that in order to be in an intimate relationship with someone I first had to learn to be separate and to have a well-developed sense of self. Otherwise, I could not let someone in without feeling overwhelmed.

Not having a well-formed sense of self can be terrifying, for it can feel like nonexistence or death. In psychology, this is referred to as narcissism. The word "narcissism" often brings to mind self-centered, self-absorbed, or self-aggrandizing, when it really means that a person has a very poorly defined sense of self and self-worth. It often goes along with a deep sense of sadness and loneliness, and it is very common in our culture, especially in people who have heart disease.

Growing up in my family, as in many families, the unspoken yet heard message from my parents was this: "You don't exist as a separate person; you are an extension of us. Therefore, you have a great capacity to cause us joy or pain. If you act right, we will be so proud of you. If you don't, we will suffer. If you really mess up, we will *really* suffer — and if we suffer enough, we will die and leave you all alone. Since you don't exist separate from us, then if we die, you'll die, too. And it will be your fault." In short, as they once wrote me, "Dean as healer, Dean as slayer." When the stakes are this high, the stresses can get very intense.

These messages have been in my family for generations. Every family has its own version of these. I'm not blaming my parents, and I love them dearly. I am deeply grateful for all they have given and done for me and the many sacrifices they have made on my behalf. They had parents and grandparents and great-grandparents who unknowingly may have given them similar messages which they unwittingly passed on to me. Each generation takes on the emotional work that wasn't completed by the previous ones.

There are many different paths to autonomy. Some are healthier than others.

One of the time-honored ways of differentiating from one's parents is to rebel, to do things they do not approve of. I found ways of rebelling that often were socially constructive — for example, taking a year off from medical school to do my first research project. "Isn't it ironic?" my parents told me in one of their more memorable moments. "You want to drop out of medical school to do research on stress and the heart and you're giving us heart attacks!" Since they didn't see me as a separate person, my behavior was often unfathomable to them.

I wanted to be in an intimate relationship, but I was afraid to be. When there are no boundaries, intimacy can feel dangerous. If you become too open to someone, you can become controlled, hurt, or even annihilated by them — often without awareness. On the other hand, being alone can be very uncomfortable for someone without a well-formed sense of self, because it feels like nonexistence. So, I found myself in relationships that were neither alone nor very intimate.

Being unmindful, I tended to choose relationships with women who also had similar issues about intimacy at that time, so we often became unhealthy mirrors for each other. As a result, I could blame *them* for not being more open or intimate without having to face my own limited capacity for intimacy then. If only *they* would change, I told myself. . . .

I remember a conversation I had twenty-five years ago with Swami Satchidananda, when I was in college, about a woman I was in love with at the time:

"She's driving me crazy!"

"Good!"

"What do you mean, 'Good!' It's not *good*, it's *horrible*."

"Why is it horrible?"

"She's doing *this*, she's not doing *that* . . . how can I get her to do *that* and not do *this?* If only she would change, then I'd be happy and everything would be wonderful."

"Look here, boy," he said, laughing compassionately. "It's not *her*, it's *you*. As long as you think the problem is with her, then you're setting yourself up for more suffering." He went on to explain that it would be empowering if I could understand that the problem was with me, because then I could do something about it. I couldn't really grasp what he meant. It took a while, but I finally began to comprehend.

This simple idea — taking responsibility and examining my own issues — was the foundation of a powerful motivational shift that began transforming my life. Before, when problems arose in a relationship, I focused on finding evidence of what the other person was doing wrong to justify and to rationalize my own habitual actions and patterns of behavior. Later, I began taking a hard look at myself and finding my own authentic response and responsibility.

When a person begins to feel accountable for his or her own actions rather than blaming the other person in the relationship, then the relationship transforms. Either the relationship may grow and become more authentic and intimate, or one person or both may decide to end a destructive relationship and choose another who is more compatible or who has a greater capacity for intimacy at that time.

As I became more aware of these patterns, I examined how I related to some people in the past. I began to feel very sorry for whatever pain I may have caused along the way. I had made some unwise choices years before that I sincerely regretted. I knew I couldn't change the past, but I became determined not to keep reliving or repeating it.

I think there is great value in living fully and making mistakes, if you survive and learn from them, because then your knowledge is authentic: it comes from your own experience. Great mistakes can lead to great wisdom, if we pay attention, learn, and stop repeating them. As William Blake wrote many years ago, "If the fool would persist in his folly, he would become wise." Robert Frost wrote, "The only way out is through."

I learned to define a separate self and to live with the terrors of facing loneliness without running from it. As a result, I could *choose* to be in one intimate relationship without the compulsion of distracting myself from real intimacy by being in several.

I have included group support sessions as part of my program since I began conducting research in reversing heart disease twenty years ago. These groups gave me the opportunity to spend extended periods of time with the same group of patients. Since the group support sessions felt increasingly safe, people became more and more self-disclosing and increasingly intimate. We got to know each other very well.

In my first study, twenty years ago, many of the men and women talked during the group support sessions about how the lack of love and intimacy in their relationships in the past may have contributed to their disease. I began to realize, Hey, that could be me in a few years if I don't make some changes in more than just diet and meditation and exercise. It's not enough to intellectually understand or to write about these issues; I need to *live* them or I might *die* them. Love and survival. How extraordinary that the people who were coming to me for healing were helping me heal myself.

What had seemed liberating — going out with different people — became increasingly frustrating. I knew that I needed to make some significant changes. The same drive that was causing these problems was now getting my attention to begin addressing them. I wanted more intimacy in my life.

I began to realize that an important part of my healing was that I needed to learn to be alone. If I wanted intimacy and love, then I first needed to learn to coexist with this pain without trying to numb it or run from it or distract myself from it in the ways that had been most familiar to me.

I spent increasing amounts of time by myself. The hardest times were when I would travel somewhere to attend a meeting or to give a lecture; afterwards, I would end up in a hotel room, alone. Unlike before, I tried not to call anyone, spend time with anyone, or even watch television or read a book in order to stay with whatever feelings arose. I discovered that when I was alone, I felt as if I were disappearing.

In one sense, I was. I was experiencing my self — more precisely, my *lack* of self — without distractions or modulation. That frightening realization helped me to begin constructing a real sense of self and self-worth.

Although it was very painful, it was healing. This same pain that I had been avoiding began cutting through some of the layers and walls that had protected my heart yet also isolated it for so many years. I began to realize that I didn't need to be with people in order to feel I existed. Slowly, little by little, my heart began to open.

While it was important for me to define a separate self as part of my own growth, it was equally important for me to go beyond separation. So much of psychotherapy tends to focus on the first half — helping people develop an autonomous, independent, separate self — at the expense of learning how to be in an intimate, sharing relationship and finding community. I am finding that real freedom comes from choosing *interdependence* rather than the false choice between codependence and independence.

I learned that the capacity for love and intimacy — an open heart — is so important to having a joyful life as well as to survival. In all relationships, not just romantic ones.

In the past, being involved with women whose capacity for intimacy at that time was as limited as my own felt safe. At least I wouldn't be controlled and consumed, even if it was frustrating because the relationship wasn't very close. As my capability for intimacy grew as a result of working on these issues, I was able to make different choices. As I began to heal, I found myself in a committed relationship with a wonderful person.

I am *not* saying that the key to happiness is finding the right Cinderella or Prince Charming, getting married, and living happily ever after. Until I had done enough work on my own obstacles to intimacy, I was incapable of being in an intimate relationship with anyone, no matter who they were. It was not about *finding* the right person; it was about *being* the right person. I knew my beloved for a long time before we got into a relationship, but I couldn't even *see* her fully at that time.

Often we don't see people for who they really are. We imagine an idealized image of them and fall in love with that, projecting that image onto the other person. As we get to know them better, we become *dis-illusioned* — quite literally, that they did not live up to our illusion of who we wanted them to be.

When I was younger, I *thought* I was in intimate relationships only because I didn't know what intimacy really meant: seeing and feeling and hearing and processing the inner world of another person instead of just projecting onto her images of who I thought she was and who I wanted her to be.

When my sweetheart and I made a commitment to the process of taking responsibility for our own behavior rather than projecting idealized images upon each other, then the possibility of real intimacy was greatly enhanced.

I began to see and to love how exquisite she really is.

This relationship is transforming my life in ways that are amazing to me. It feels like grace. Through it, I have learned how to experience happiness on a different level. Not all the time, of course, but with much greater continuity and depth than before. The more whole I feel within myself, the greater the capacity I have for intimacy with someone else.

The great scientist Louis Pasteur once wrote, "Chance favors the prepared mind." I believe that grace favors an open heart. More precisely, grace *is* an open heart.

When you "fall in love," it is usually with your illusion, your projection; it is not the same as opening your heart to your beloved. To paraphrase the author Henry Miller, I don't think I can fall in love again, so now maybe I can really learn to love someone. This idea is beautifully expressed in Psalm 1 of the book of Psalms, translated by Stephen Mitchell:

Blessed are the man and the woman
who have grown beyond their greed
and have put an end to their hatred
and no longer nourish illusions.
But they delight in the way things are
and keep their hearts open, day and night.
They are like trees planted near flowing rivers,
which bear fruit when they are ready.
Their leaves will not fall or wither.
Everything they do will succeed.

When two people commit themselves to each other, magic can begin to happen. Instead of repeating the same superficial experience with different people, I am having different, extraordinary experiences with the same person.

More than a hundred years ago, Ramakrishna talked about the importance of making a commitment to one spiritual teacher or tradition and following that path rather than going from one teacher to another. You can dig one deep well and reach a wellspring of water or you can drill a hundred shallow, dry ones. The same is true in other relationships.

I had realized long before that great sex is no substitute for an open heart. What I began learning is that an open heart can lead to the most joyful and ecstatic sex. Every day, my beloved and I are learning to trust each other a little more so the walls around our hearts begin opening a little further. All the clichés come to mind — our hearts opening wider and wider, like layers of an onion being peeled away. I realize how wonderful it feels to be truly relaxed and comfortable with another person.

Guitarist Tuck Andress and singer Patti Cathcart are extraordinary musicians whose music is both powerful and loving. They are also married to each other. I once heard Tuck describing their relationship.

My life's work is to subsume my ego into this greater whole, both musically and in our personal relationship. I spent so many years becoming a great guitar technician, practicing alone. It was a real change for me to play with someone else, learning how to listen, how to hear through her ears.

I've spent time just learning how to play one note, over and over. We've played some songs thousands of times, but there's always something fresh and new to find there. Just like our relationship. If it becomes stale, then I dig more deeply into the rut, I don't abandon it. To find the freshness that's there. The universe is right here, not over there. To leave room and space for the magic. There is the same level of detail at any level of magnification, from the subatomic to the universal, if you look closely enough.

Commitment in relationship can lead to real freedom and joy. By analogy, the same is as true of diet as it is of relationships. Many people have said to me over the years, "I could never change my diet. I want to *enjoy* what I eat." To me, there is no point in giving up something I enjoy unless I get something back that's even better. And quickly.

I began eating a low-fat vegetarian diet when I was nineteen, not because I was worried about my heart or my health or living to be one hundred. I did it because I found I felt so much better. More energy. Less sleep. A greater sense of well-being.

People with heart disease generally notice marked improvements in the frequency of angina (chest pain). Someone who can't work, or walk, or make love, or even shower or shave without getting chest pain often finds that he or she can begin to do all of these activities a few weeks after changing the diet — if the changes are big enough. This reframes the reason for changing from fear of dying to joy of living. You don't have to wait thirty years for the benefit. Many people now prefer the taste of healthy, low-fat foods.

One of the most effective antismoking ad campaigns asked, "Do you want to taste like an ashtray to your lover?" Kissing is more fun than smoking. It was much more powerful than asking, "Do you want to get lung cancer?" because the benefits of kissing are much more real and immediate than the threat of cancer, which is in the future and too terrifying to think about.

In a similar way, I am finding that being in a committed, monogamous relationship has given me more joy and freedom than ever. The act of making a commitment itself has value, in relationships as well as in diet.

All religions have dietary restrictions, but they differ from one to another. One religion allows you to eat certain foods that are forbidden in another. I don't think God is confused, nor are we. Whatever the intrinsic benefit in eating or not eating certain foods, just the act of choosing not to eat or not to do something helps to make our lives more sacred, more special.

In other words, we may choose to follow the restrictions of our own religion or tradition not to *please* God but rather to *experience* God. We begin to heal our separation from God and from each other. Also, choosing *not* to do something helps us define who we are. A person without a separate self has no real choice. Freedom comes from choosing *not* to do something as well as from choosing to *do* something. Only when we can say no are we free to say yes.

In a committed relationship, saying no to everyone but your beloved sanctifies the relationship. Not in the dry, boring sense — rather, *sacred* is just another way of saying *the most special,* which, in turn, makes it the most fun, the most joyful, the most wonderful.

Of course, relationships can be stultifying and oppressive. Some people experience religious or dietary restrictions in a similar way. Whether or not discipline, monogamy, and commitment are liberating or confining is in part a function of whether or not you feel free to choose or whether these are imposed on you.

When I can see and love God in my beloved, and then in myself, then I can begin to love and see and experience God in everyone and everything. I am learning that the sacred is found not just in altars of churches and synagogues, not just by looking for the extraordinary, but rather by finding the extraordinary in the ordinary — thereby removing barriers that separate us from each other and from ourselves.

Sitting on the couch watching a movie, eating popcorn, going for a walk together, holding hands, watching her sleep, kissing, sharing a meal together. Somehow, these simple moments are far more meaningful to me than any award or accomplishment. As in the television show *Seinfeld,* life's everyday experiences also can be the most fun.

An appreciative patient told me recently, "I want to thank you in all the languages known." When I came home, I told my sweetheart, "I want to say I love you in all the languages known."

"How about Braille?" she replied.

For so much of my life, I felt as if I had to show that I was special by doing extraordinary things in order to be loved. This approach was self-defeating, for to be special in that way was to be isolated, different — setting myself apart from others in hopes that would help me feel close to them. I began to learn that those who really loved me did so *despite* what I've done, not because of it. Others may have become envious, causing even more separation and isolation.

I used to feel loved because I was special. Now, I feel special because I am loved and because I *can* love. We all have the ability to love, to be loved, and, thus, to feel special.

I'm learning that the real grace is not just being loved; it is learning how to love. I have needed trust, commitment, and complete honesty in order to feel safe enough to make myself vulnerable to love someone else without holding back. In this context, commitment can be liberating.

In the movie *City Slickers*, the character played by Billy Crystal is asked by his friend, also a married man, "Let's say a spaceship lands and the most beautiful woman you ever saw gets out. All she wants to do is have the greatest sex in the universe with you. And the second it's over, she flies away for eternity. No one will ever know. And you're telling me you wouldn't do it?"

"No. What you're describing actually happened to my cousin Ronald. And his wife *did* find out about it at the beauty parlor. They know *everything* there."

"Forget about it!"

"Look, Ed, what I'm saying is it wouldn't make it all right if Barbara didn't know. *I'd* know. And I wouldn't like myself. That's all."

I know a married couple who were having intimacy problems. The man seriously considered having an affair with a woman he had known for a while. He said he didn't tell his wife about his frustrations because he was afraid that knowing about these feelings might hurt her and make their intimacy problems even worse.

"This can become a self-fulfilling prophecy. Some part of her already knows," I said to him. "At some level, we are all interconnected. Thus, every lie is known at some level, even if the other person does not consciously want to acknowledge it. Every lie to your loved one, every deceit — no matter how seemingly small or trivial — causes trust to begin dying. As trust dies, intimacy withers.

"If you don't tell her, she may begin to wall herself off from you out of fear of being hurt. You may find yourself fighting about things that seem to make no sense, because that's not what the arguments are really about. If that happens, you will probably become increasingly frustrated by the arguments and the lack of intimacy. The new woman will then seem even more appealing (she knows the secret, but your wife does not), and you'll feel more and more justified in being with her, perhaps even sleeping with her, which creates an even bigger secret and an even bigger wall.

"But the new woman can't trust you, either, because she knows you haven't been honest with your wife, so the ability to be intimate with the new woman is also limited. As a result, you may find yourself becoming increasingly frustrated by the limitations of intimacy with the new woman just as you were with your wife, and you're back where you started. Lonely. There is a verse from the *I Ching*: 'Three becomes two becomes one.'

"Instead, you could try being completely honest with your wife about your feelings. It may be painful at first, but at least you have the possibility of real intimacy. Or, you may find after careful consideration and working on the relationship that it's not the right one for you. If so, you could end the relationship with integrity and on healthier and more amicable terms than if you betray your wife's trust. Also, you have the possibility of greater intimacy if you go into another relation-ship."

He decided to tell his wife the truth about what he was feeling. It *was* very painful for both of them at first. They went into couples counseling together. Now, the relationship is far more intimate and they are much happier than ever before. Of course, they still have disagreements, but they now have a way of discussing and resolving these issues rather than ignoring or acting them out in destructive ways.

As I learn how to open my heart to my beloved, I have moments when I actually feel love for myself. Not in a narcissistic way (it's hard to love yourself if you don't *have* a self), but in a way that feels whole, holy, and healing. The more love I feel for myself, the more love I have to give others.

As I feel more compassion for myself, I have a greater capacity to view others with more compassion and with less judgment. At times, I can experience the transcendent interconnectedness — the universal Self, which goes by many names and forms — without getting lost in it, maintaining a "double vision" of the oneness *and* the diversity. I can sometimes see the chessboard and the various pieces, each with its own role, and I can also see the wood from which the board and all of the chess pieces were carved.

Several thousand years ago, the Egyptian philosopher Hermes Trismegistus wrote, "As above, so below." We can unite the sacred and profane, the inner and outer, the spiritual and worldly, the transcendent God and the God within ourselves.

From that perspective, we can begin to love our neighbor *as* our Self in different forms — which is the essence of empathy and compassion. As the American poet Walt Whitman wrote in 1855 in his masterwork, *Leaves of Grass*, "I do not ask how the wounded one feels; I, myself, *become* the wounded one." More on this in chapter 4.

Some very old wounds began healing. This is a long way from wanting to commit suicide at age nineteen.

Your Lifestyle Hasn't Caught Up with Your Life

Feelings of trust, vulnerability, and intimacy I have found so healing in my personal life are a powerful force in my work with others. When people attend one of the residential retreats my colleagues and I offer, most of them tend to view the group support sessions as perhaps the least important part

163

of my program in the beginning. By the end of the week — and often by the end of the first day — they often view the group support as the most meaningful part of what we do. It nurtures their spirit in the same way that food nourishes their bodies. I will describe our group process more thoroughly in chapter 4.

For a while, I was neither here nor there, halfway out the door — like the proverbial monkey who has its hand stuck in the cookie jar and needs to let go of the cookie to get his hand out of the jar. I realized it, but I didn't want to let go of the cookie.

But I am making progress. If I believe that my relationship with my beloved is the most meaningful and important aspect of my life — and I do — then I need to act that way.

Someone once told me that how you spend your time says a lot more about what you really value than anything you might say is important to you. I began to realize that if I really value this relationship, then I needed to act accordingly. It caused me to change how I spend my time. I am learning to say no to a lot of cookies.

I was offered an extraordinary work opportunity, something I used to dream about earlier in my career. It would have meant working even harder than I did for several more years. I lost a lot of sleep over whether or not I should accept this — until one day I had the following conversation with my friend Rachel, who has known me for a long time. After patiently listening to me run in the same circles for the fourth time, she challenged me:

Rachel: Let me just cut to the chase here: Why aren't you listening to yourself? What allows your soul to flourish?

Dean: Love and joy.

Rachel: Your joy is the marker for what's right for you. Joy comes from connecting to your soul's purpose. Will this new opportunity bring you more joy than having more time for your relationship and starting a family?

Dean: No, but it is such a golden opportunity.

Rachel: If you are swimming in the ocean and someone offers you a great big bag of gold — a golden opportunity — if you take that bag and hold on to it, you will drown. Are you going to hold on to something that will keep you from what most nourishes your soul? Either you let go now or you become a slave to the very thing you created and it tells you how to live. Now, you have someone real in your life and you won't have time to go home and see her. Your lifestyle hasn't caught up with your life!

I began to understand that the choice is not between working and not working, accomplishing or not accomplishing; it is the intentionality behind the action, not the action itself, that determines whether it leads to healing and joy or suffering and illness. One of my favorite Zen proverbs states, "Before enlightenment, chop wood, carry water; after enlightenment, chop wood, carry water." The actions may look the same, the work may be hard, but the motivation can be quite different.

If the intention behind the work is to seek recognition and power — "Hey, look at me, I'm *special,* I'm *important,* I'm worthy of your love and respect" — then you are setting yourself apart from others as a way of trying to feel connected to them. *Setting yourself apart from others as a way of trying to feel connected to them:* It seems so clear why this is self-defeating, and yet it is often the norm in our culture. But the norm is not normal.

Investing not only your self-worth but even your sense of self in the outcome of what you do is a very high-stakes game. It's not just winning or losing; it's being a winner or loser. Winners are loved, losers are lonely, so the stakes and the stresses become very high. Or so we believe.

There is another intention for doing work: "I love and I feel loved. I do this work as an expression of love and service. I am loved for who I *am*, not for what I *do* or for what I *have*." Although the work may seem the same, the effects are strikingly different.

Actions performed with this motivation lead to wholeness and healing, not isolation and suffering. There is much less anxiety and attachment to the outcome because the stakes are quite different. Because of this, paradoxically, the quality of the work may be much greater.

It becomes easier to make balanced choices when I don't feel compelled to take an opportunity because it will look good on my résumé. Before, in a very real sense, I didn't even have a choice. When my self-worth was defined by what I did, then I had to take every important opportunity that came along, even if relationships suffered. Now I understand that real power is measured not by how much you have but rather by how much you can walk away from.

In an interview, the actor Ralph Fiennes (*The English Patient*) was asked, "Don't fame and success isolate you from what you were before and from those you loved?" He replied:

> "Success?" Fiennes gave me a withering look. "Well, I don't know quite what you mean by success. Material success? Worldly success? Personal, emotional success? The people I consider successful are so because of how they handle their responsibilities to other people, how they approach the future, people who have a full sense of the value of their life and what they want to do with it.
>
> "I call people 'successful' not because they have money or their business is doing well but because, as human beings, they have a fully developed sense of being alive and engaged in a lifetime task of collaboration with other human beings — their mothers and fathers, their family, their friends, their loved ones, the friends who are dying, the friends who are being born.

"Success?" he repeated emphatically. "Don't you know it is all about being able to extend love to people? Not in a big, capital-letter sense but in the everyday. Little by little, task by task, gesture by gesture, word by word."

For me, learning how to open my heart and be intimate with another person continues to be a powerful, healing experience. Of course, this is only one of many pathways to healing and intimacy. In chapter 4, I will describe several approaches that you may find helpful.

I am learning that the key to our survival is love. When we love someone and feel loved by them, somehow along the way our suffering subsides, our deepest wounds begin healing, our hearts start to feel safe enough to be vulnerable and to open a little wider. We begin experiencing our own emotions and the feelings of those around us.

Dr. George Wald, a Harvard biologist who won the Nobel Prize, once wrote, "What one really needs is not Nobel laureates but love. How do you think one gets to be a Nobel laureate? Wanting love, that's how. Wanting it so bad one works all the time and ends up a Nobel laureate. It's a consolation prize. What matters is love."

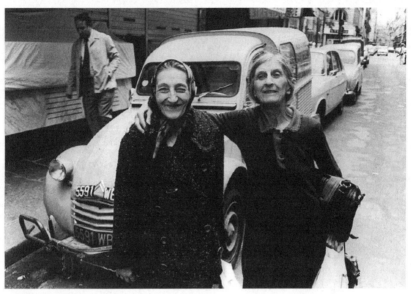

Paris, 1974

<h1 style="text-align:center">4</h1>

Pathways to Love
and Intimacy

There are many pathways to love and intimacy. In the continuing process of learning to open my heart, I have found some paths that have been very helpful to me. Here are a few of them. This is by no means a complete list, only an overview. Many of the patients with whom I have worked also have benefited greatly from these methods.

The previous chapter described my own ongoing process in learning how to live more fully. However, a romantic relationship is only one of countless ways of experiencing the healing power of love and intimacy. In this chapter, I will explore some other strategies for enhancing and facilitating love and intimacy.

This is not a how-to book; rather, it is a *what-if* book: an exploration of the powerful roles love and intimacy play in our survival. What if we make different choices?

Many wonderful books have been written about communication skills, about meditation, about a variety of other ways to increase intimacy in your life. As I wrote earlier, awareness is the first step in healing. If I have succeeded in clarifying why love and intimacy are so important, then I hope this will inspire you in your own explorations. This chapter is only a taste of the feast that lies before you. If you have the intention to learn more, you may find a wealth of information available to you that may previously have gone unnoticed.

The journey to greater love and intimacy is perhaps the most personal and meaningful of all life's adventures. Traveling your own path is more valuable than following in someone else's footsteps, although we can all learn from the experiences of others. As Carlos Castaneda wrote in *The Teachings of Don Juan*,

> Before you embark on it you ask the question: Does this path have a heart? If the answer is no, you will know it, and then you must choose another path. . . . A path without a heart is never enjoyable. You have to work hard even to take it. On the other hand, a path with heart is easy; it does not make you work at liking it.

If your awareness is present and your intention is focused, then you will find your own way. Resources, books, teachers, events, guides, and information may become available to you in ways that might seem mysterious or even magical. In part, this is a function of your own heightened awareness: You are more likely to see what you are looking for. If you are hungry and drive down the street, you will probably observe the restaurants and not even notice the gas stations, but if your fuel tank is low, you may be more likely to see the gas stations and ignore the restaurants. We only see a fraction of what is right in front of us. For example, do you remember what framed picture was hanging on the wall at the last hotel in which you stayed?

Yet more is going on than just heightened awareness. There is also grace. If you make a commitment to your journey of the heart, forces come into play that are part of life's mystery. "Ask, and it will be given to you; seek, and you will find; knock, and the door will be opened to you. For everyone who asks, receives; and he who seeks, finds; and to him who knocks, the door will be opened" (Matthew 7:7). I don't pretend to understand why, but I have seen it time and time again in my own life and in the lives of others. Teachers come in many forms and disguises.

You may want to find a teacher, or you may prefer to do it on your own. You may already draw strength and wisdom from your own religion, or you may find yourself investigating other ones — or, as in my case, you may discover new meaning and value in your own religion after exploring the rich spiritual traditions of others. You might prefer a secular approach. Although the techniques and approaches all vary in their form and style, the underlying theme and purpose remains the same: Anything that promotes intimacy leads to greater joy and healing; anything that promotes isolation and loneliness leads to more suffering and illness.

Techniques can be useful, but they are limited. I am finding that I have a choice in every moment to keep my heart open or closed, to live in love or in fear. More than any specific practice, I have found that maintaining this awareness of choice is the most important factor in keeping an open heart, for every action, every thought, every moment contains the potential for bringing us closer to either intimacy and healing or isolation and suffering. The direction is not inherent in the actions themselves but rather in the intentionality and motivation behind the actions.

The same hand that caresses also can kill. The same voice that soothes also can attack. Sexual intercourse can be an expression of deep love and a return to the source of transcendent union and oneness or, in the case of rape, it can be one of life's most isolating and destructive experiences. Millard Fuller is the visionary founder of Habitat for Humanity, which has constructed homes for hundreds of thousands of homeless people worldwide. In his book *The Theology of the Hammer*, he writes about how the same hammer that nailed Jesus to the cross can be used to build and renovate homes for those in need.

When the intentionality and motivation are an open heart, then our actions tend to move us closer to intimacy and healing rather than isolation and suffering. As Swami Satchidananda has written:

> Spiritual practice is not what you are *doing*, but what you are *thinking*: what is the motivation for your actions? You don't have to change your activities and say, "This is spiritual practice but this is not." Even when you sit on the toilet you are doing spiritual practice if you have the right intention. We should transform all our activities into spiritual practice. That means, "I am doing everything as a meditation, as an offering, as a prayer to serve God through service to humanity."

In other words, when you eat, you might remind yourself, "I am eating not only to enjoy the food and nourish my body, but also so I can stay strong and healthy in order to help other people." That same attitude of service can transform worldly activities into spiritual ones.

Similarly, technology has the potential to

bring us closer together or to isolate us further. As with everything, it is not technology in and of itself, but rather how we use it. The explosive growth of interactive computer networks such as America Online, Compuserve, the Well, and others is due in large part to the chat rooms and opportunities for "virtual community" that they provide. At their best, E-mail and chat rooms can be another way of staying in touch and keeping up with loved ones who may be thousands of miles away in real space but instantly available in cyberspace. All too often, however, technology provides a way of numbing loneliness without experiencing real intimacy.

Sherry Turkle was on the faculty of the Massachusetts Institute of Technology's program in Science, Technology and Society when she wrote:

Terrified of being alone, yet afraid of intimacy, we experience widespread feelings of emptiness, of disconnection, of the unreality of self. And here the computer, a companion without emotional demands, offers a compromise. You can be a loner, but never alone. You can interact, but need never feel vulnerable to another person.

Yet the willingness to feel vulnerable — to open your heart — is essential to real intimacy. Communication is a fundamental skill for building connection and contact, communion and community. Let's begin with communication skills, which are based on choosing to make ourselves vulnerable to another person as a way of feeling closer to them.

Words Matter

What we say — and how we say it — can have a powerful effect on bringing us closer to or farther from another person.

Let me begin with an example that I often use when I lecture. This exercise needs at least two people: one to read it, and at least one to listen.

> **Reader**: Close your eyes. Take a deep breath. Get comfortable. Center yourself. Pay attention to how you feel when I say what I am about to express:
> "I think you are *wrong!* And I think you're a *jerk!*"
> OK. Open your eyes. How did that feel? Notice all the feelings and sensations that you experienced in that moment.

Most people report that they don't feel

very good. You might feel angry. Attacked. Criticized. Judged. Shamed. Upset. Hostile. Combative. Depressed. You may experience pressure or tightness in your chest, your jaw, your back, your stomach, or shoulders.

This sense of tightness, constriction, and closing down is a physiological response — your muscles constrict, even your arteries may constrict — as well as an emotional and even a metaphorical one: constriction and withdrawal of yourself from others as a way of trying to protect yourself physically and emotionally. You may even have stopped breathing for a moment.

In this example, would you want to get to know the reader better in that moment? Probably not. Did you want to know why he or she thought you were wrong or why he or she thought you were a jerk? Probably not. Did you feel attacked or judged? Probably so. If this were real life, what would you want to do next?

We often think of ourselves as complex human beings with an infinite range of human responses. In reality, most people respond to feeling attacked or judged in one of two basic ways:

- withdraw
- attack

You can withdraw in many ways. One way is to withdraw physically, to leave the room — "Later for you!" If you can't leave the room — out of fear of the repercussions or because the other person has more power than you, for example — then you may just withdraw mentally. You zone out; you are not there anymore. Either way, the wall around your heart says, "You see, I *told* you it wasn't safe," and the wall just grows thicker and more fortified.

If you attack back and say, "No, *you* are a jerk and *you're* the one who's wrong," then the other person usually attacks back and the situation tends to spiral downward, often escalating from there.

Intimacy is the first casualty of attacking or withdrawing. To the degree that the lack of intimacy affects our quality of life, our health, and even our survival, then we are putting each of these in jeopardy when we communicate in this manner.

There is another way.

Reader: Close your eyes again. Take a deep breath. Get comfortable. Center yourself. Pay attention to how you feel when I say what I am about to express: "I feel angry. I feel upset."

OK. Open your eyes again. Was it the

same or different. Notice all the feelings and sensations that you experienced in that moment.

Most people find this to be a very different experience. You may be curious to want to know more about why I feel that way. You are drawn into wanting to find out why I am angry and upset. You are less likely to feel that same tightness and constriction in your throat, chest, or stomach. You are much less likely to feel judged or attacked or criticized, so there is much less need to withdraw or attack back.

This is not about making nice. This is not about the power of positive thinking. *This is about being real and authentic.*

It may seem that both examples are about being real. If I say, "I think you're a jerk," that's real. If I say, "I'm angry," that's also real. Why is the impact so different?

The first example is a thought. The second example is a feeling.

We tend to hear thoughts as judgments and criticisms, which close the heart. We tend to hear feelings in a very different way, with an open heart — as an invitation to move closer together, a sense of openness. Our feelings connect us with each other.

Now, it may have sounded like semantics

until you experienced the difference. This example wasn't even real life. You know this is just an exercise, and yet even so, at a visceral level, you probably felt the effects, for better and for worse. The words that we use really do matter. They matter to other people, and they matter to us.

Why are feelings more likely to be heard and less likely to be perceived as attacks than thoughts?

When we express our feelings, we make ourselves more vulnerable. When we make ourselves vulnerable, it becomes safer for the other person to do so as well. As we discussed, we can experience intimacy only to the degree that we are willing to risk being vulnerable. Hearts that are open feel connected to each other.

It can be frightening to make yourself vulnerable to another person — because you might get hurt. The commitment of a long-term relationship can help both people feel safer and thus more willing to be vulnerable. Such vulnerability, however, is a double-edged sword: You know each other's soft spots when you are in a relationship with someone, so no one can hurt you as efficiently or as badly as your beloved, who knows your soft underbelly, just where to zing you.

That is the dilemma. You can't really be in an intimate relationship without being vulnerable, but when you feel attacked, the last thing you want to do is to make yourself vulnerable. When you feel judged or criticized or attacked, you stop listening. Then the aspects that make a relationship the most joyful are the ones that become the most painful. Over time, you may even begin to feel like it's not even worth getting into it because it hurts too much: "Let's just keep it safe and numb." It's not too intimate, it's not too fulfilling, but at least it's better than feeling that kind of pain. Or, in some extremes, leading parallel lives where the people are there together in body, but not really in spirit, which is not really very fulfilling.

It doesn't just stop there. Relationships are also about balancing and sharing power. When one person feels attacked or judged, he or she feels disempowered and perceives a power imbalance. One person feels one-up, and the other feels one-down. When that happens, the person feeling disempowered usually finds a way to reempower himself or herself. This can play out in a number of different ways.

Maybe the next time you want to have sex, the other person will not be interested. Or maybe the next time you want to go somewhere, the other person doesn't want to go. Maybe that person won't even tell you the real reason. It's just, "Oh, I don't feel good tonight, honey." Or "I don't really want to go there" or "I'm really busy. I need to work late at the office tonight." When a person feels criticized, it makes it difficult for him or her to give you what you want, even if the person would otherwise want to do so.

It is painful to feel attacked by your beloved, and it is equally painful if he or she withdraws from you:

"I can see you are angry; let's talk about it. How are you doing?"

"No, everything is fine," is the reply, yet you can feel the anger there.

If someone doesn't feel strong enough to be aggressive or assertive, then he or she might act passive-aggressive and withholding. Either accomplishes the same goal of redressing perceived power imbalances.

Why would people want to do that? They are reacting to a perceived attack or judgment in the only way that they know how. These are very common ways of relating, but they are not fun, nor in our own best interests.

I have learned from making many painful mistakes that almost nothing in my life brings me as much joy and pleasure as feeling close with my beloved. I have also learned how quickly criticism can impede this feeling of intimacy. In the past, I was quick to criticize. Now, it has to be something very important for me to say anything critical to my beloved, for few issues are worth disturbing that wonderful feeling of closeness.

We both want to be in an authentic relationship, yet we don't want to disturb the closeness. How do we manage to communicate real feelings without interfering with intimacy?

Communicating real feelings *is* intimate. When we communicate feelings — as real feelings rather than as thoughts — then we can be authentic *and* intimate.

It's not that feelings are better than thoughts. After all, I make my living by thinking. It's knowing when each is more effective. "I think you did a great job" is a thought. If you are supervising somebody, it may be appropriate to give them your thoughts and judgments. Just be aware of the impact of them.

There is great power in authenticity. If you say, "Gee, everything is fine" when it isn't, then there is a disconnect between what you are really feeling and what you are expressing. At some level, when you are inauthentic with yourself and with others, it is a betrayal of your own integrity and your own body, your own immune system, your own cardiovascular system. At some level, your body knows that.

In the movie *Liar Liar*, the character played by Jim Carrey is forced to speak only the truth for one day. It's funny to watch how hard it is for him to do that. It made me think: How many times during the day do we not speak our own truth? How many times a day do we say something that isn't completely authentic?

When you are authentic with yourself and with others, then you have integrity. When you have integrity, you have greater personal power, charisma, and authority, all of which can be felt by you and by those around you.

It is difficult to be authentic if the choice seems to be, "Well, if I tell him that he's a jerk, then I'm going to get in a fight with him or he's going to withdraw, so I am not going to feel good about that. If I don't say anything, then I am not going to feel good about that, either." So, after a while, many people learn to suppress their feelings if they don't know what to do with them.

There is another strategy here, which is to be authentic but to express your feelings rather than thoughts. It's about speaking your truth to someone in a way that he or she is more likely to hear without feeling judged or criticized. Learning a few basic communication skills can make a profound difference in how intimate and connected we feel with other people. These skills are worth learning and worth practicing even though they don't come naturally for most of us.

The first step is to understand the difference between a thought and a feeling.

Some examples of thoughts:

I think you're wrong.
I feel that you're wrong.

Wait a minute! "I feel that you're wrong" is a feeling, right?

No. When you say, "I feel that . . . ," this is usually a thought masquerading as a feeling. It's still a judgment. So are expressions like "I feel like you should. . . ." or "I feel like you are. . . ." Expressions such as "you always," "you never," "you should," and "you ought to" are almost always heard as criticisms and judgments.

Some examples of feelings:

I feel hurt.
I feel angry.
I feel upset.

I feel worried.
I feel unloved and unappreciated.
I feel good.
I feel happy.
I feel alone.
I feel scared.
I feel anxious.
I feel aroused and sexual.
I feel bad.
I feel sick.
I feel healthy.

You get the idea.

Saying, "I want" is also a feeling. Sometimes we avoid saying "I want" because on the surface it seems too direct or even demanding and may seem inappropriate. In reality, though, I think that we may be reluctant to say "I want" because it makes us vulnerable. As I wrote earlier, sharing feelings makes us vulnerable — which is why it works to make us more intimate. If you say, "I want _____," someone, in effect, now has the power to make you unhappy or happy, at least within this context, depending on whether or not they give it to you.

In some cultures, especially in Asian countries, it is considered socially impolite to say, "I want _____." I used to think they were more circumspect because saying "I want" was too direct. Now, I understand that their reserve is also a way of saving face by not making oneself vulnerable. You would lose face if you said that you wanted something and then did not get it.

In a healthy relationship, you often want to give the other person what he or she wants. It makes you happy to please your partner, even if it is inconvenient for you. As soon as you feel attacked or judged, however, the last thing in the world you want to do is make your partner happy, even if otherwise you would have been willing to give them what they want.

So, whether for selfish reasons or for unselfish ones, expressing your feelings is more likely to get what you want. Even when you don't get what you want, you preserve the intimacy, which is even more precious.

There are many other reasons why feelings are less likely to be heard as judgments or attacks than thoughts.

Feelings are true. Thoughts can be argued about. When you tell me what you are feeling, that is your experience. I can't argue with you. I can't say, "No, you're really not feeling that way," because the only person who knows how you feel is you. If you say, "I think you're a jerk," then we can argue about whether or not I really am. If you say,

"I feel angry," then that is a true statement by definition. Then I can wonder, "Why are you feeling that way?" which is the beginning of a real dialogue.

Feelings keep us in the present moment, where infinite possibilities exist. Thoughts keep us stuck in the past. "Well, you've always been a jerk. Not only are you a jerk today, you were a jerk before." In the present moment, anything is possible. Just because we may have acted or reacted in similar ways in the past doesn't mean we have to keep doing so. We can do it differently now.

Emotions influence us more than thoughts. Thoughts are processed and filtered in your head; feelings go straight to your heart. Some of the most successful movie producers have told me that they almost always strive for the scenes that evoke feelings rather than thoughts. Advertisements, political and fund-raising campaigns, propaganda — in other words, systematic efforts to influence your behavior — are much more likely to appeal to your emotions than to rational discourse because they work more effectively.

The ability to feel another's emotions is the essence of compassion. When we express what we are really feeling to another, we offer them the gift of understanding. I will describe this process further in the next section.

In summary, here are some key points for improving communication to enhance love and intimacy:

- **_Identify what you are feeling._** What you are _really_ feeling, not what you believe you ought to feel. This can be harder than it sounds. It takes practice. Part of the value of quieting your mind with meditation or prayer is that it can help you pay greater attention to what you're really feeling. For example, in the middle of an intense discussion I often ask myself, "What am I really feeling now?" Paying attention to your emotions also can be a clue to what another person is feeling. Hearts tend to resonate with each other. When I studied psychiatry as part of my general internal medicine residency, I was trained to pay attention to what I felt when a patient first entered the room as a clue to what that patient might be experiencing. For example, if I suddenly began to feel a little depressed or angry or happy when a patient walked in, chances are that person might also be having those feelings.
- **_Disclose what you are feeling._** Tell the other person directly and clearly what and how you are feeling. Be careful

to express your feelings, not your thoughts.

- **Listen carefully to what the other person is feeling.** If they express thoughts and judgments, you may wish to avoid getting caught in the trap of attack/withdraw/counterattack. You have other choices. If you feel judged, you might express: "I'm feeling attacked and judged, and I don't like it." The other person may not be as aware of communication skills, so you can elicit and probe for what the other person is feeling: "I'm interested in what you're feeling about this."
- **Acknowledge the other person's feelings, with empathy, caring, and compassion.** It can be helpful to repeat back to the other person a summary of what you've heard. "I understand that you're upset and you want me to be on time. I'm sorry for having inconvenienced you and I will do my best to be on time in the future."

Let me give an example from one of the weeklong residential retreats that my colleagues and I offer four times per year through our nonprofit research institute. After I give a lecture on these communication skills, I ask for a couple to volunteer to re-enact a fight or a misunderstanding that they had. Along the way, I point out when each person is saying something that is likely to be heard as an attack or judgment by the other person, and then ask the other person to explain how they reacted when they felt attacked or judged. Then I ask each person to redo the dialogue using the communication skills described here and to notice how much closer and more intimate they feel.

Below is an example from one of these retreats. I deliberately chose one in which the couple is arguing over something relatively trivial, for it is these common, day-to-day disagreements that are often the most frustrating.

Dean: I need two people who are in a relationship with each other to re-enact a recent argument in front of the group. Both members of the couple have to be willing to do this. Any volunteers?

[Bob and Carol volunteer.]

Dean: Thank you. Welcome. What I would like you to do is to reenact the quarrel now. Then we will redo it in ways that may be easier for each of you to hear what the other is saying and feeling. So, who wants to start?

Bob: Go ahead, Carol.

Carol: Bob, I picked up your messages today.

Bob: How come you did that?

Carol: Well, I am trying to help you.

Bob: You don't need to do that.

Carol: I don't need to help you?

Bob: I like to hear my messages first-hand.

Carol: But I'm just being thoughtful. I wrote them all down. Did you read them?

Bob: No.

Carol: See, I spend all this time trying to help you and assist you and to ease your life, ease your stress, and you don't appreciate me!

Bob: Well, that doesn't save me any time! When I come in, I want to pick up my own messages, listen to them myself. I want to hear that voice. I want to know the tone of the person's voice.

Carol: Okay. Fine. You do it yourself. [*At that point, Carol said she started to leave the room.*]

Bob: Well, you don't need to do that. I didn't mean it that way.

Carol:	You don't need me to help you. Fine.
Bob:	No. I need you. Come back here. Come back here! I want to talk to you!
Carol:	This is how it goes.
Dean:	Okay. Does that sound at all familiar to anybody?
Audience:	Yes.
Dean:	Okay. Now, after that exchange happened, did you feel closer to each other?
Carol:	No!
Dean:	Bob, did you feel closer to Carol?
Bob:	No. I felt a distance there. It didn't feel good.
Dean:	Okay. Now, can you remember a time when you felt really connected to Carol? And Carol, can you remember a time when you felt really connected to Bob?
Carol:	Yes. It felt wonderful.
Dean:	Is there anything in life that feels better to you?
Carol:	No.
Dean:	Bob, is there anything that feels better to you?
Bob:	No.
Dean:	Okay. So, when we stop and think about it, there is almost

nothing that is worth jeopardizing that feeling of intimacy and closeness.

Carol: That's right.

Bob: I agree.

Dean: On the other hand, at the end of this quarrel, you felt like you didn't want to be around that person for a while. And that feels pretty bad.

Bob: Right.

Carol: I felt very alone. And there are not a lot of things that feel as bad as that.

Bob: Yeah. You don't feel the oneness.

Dean: On the one hand, you have a feeling that is better than just about anything — if not the best. On the other hand, you have a feeling that is just about worse than anything — if not the worst. So, if we are being logical about it, we might say, "You know, there are not many things that are really worth going from feeling so good to feeling so bad." I doubt that this was important enough to be worth jeopardizing the intimacy in your relationship.

Carol: That's right.

Bob: Right.

Dean: And yet, we may do it over and over and over again. Why? Because we don't think about it, because we are in these patterns, because it's familiar: We have other choices. So let's try it differently. What I want you to do is think about the feelings that come up for you at each moment along the way, and to express them as feelings. Okay?

Carol: Okay.

Dean: So, let's try it again. Let's rewind the mental video and let's go back to where we started. Bob, I want you to imagine that you are in real time back when this argument happened and remember what you were really feeling when she said that she picked up your messages.

Carol: Bob, I picked up your messages today.

Dean: Now stop here. What are you feeling when she says that?

Bob: I felt like she invaded my privacy to a certain extent.

Dean: If you say "I feel like . . ." or "I feel that . . . ," that is actually a thought. What is the feeling be-

	hind that? You could say, "I feel invaded," if that's how you felt.
Bob:	I felt invaded. I didn't appreciate her picking up my messages, really.
Dean:	Okay. What else? What other feelings?
Bob:	Frustration and anger.
Dean:	Okay. So, express whatever you feel now to Carol.
Bob:	Carol, I feel that you made me angry and frustrated.
Dean:	Those are thoughts masquerading as feelings. They are likely to be heard as judgments and blame.
Carol:	Exactly. I wanted to run away when he said that.
Dean:	So, Bob, what do you feel? You see, it's not easy; it takes practice.
Bob:	I feel you shouldn't have picked up my messages.
Dean:	Is "I feel that you shouldn't have picked up my messages" a thought or a feeling?
Audience:	: A thought.
Dean:	Yes. It's a judgment. You didn't say it, but the word *that* was implied. What is the feeling behind

	that? We just talked about some of these — you said you felt invaded, frustrated, and angry. You might share those feelings with Carol.
Bob:	Carol, I feel invaded, frustrated, and angry when you pick up my messages.
Dean:	Stop there. Now, when he says that, do you feel attacked in that moment?
Carol:	No.
Dean:	It's a different experience. What are you feeling now?
Carol:	Well, I feel . . . I feel like apologizing to him.
Dean:	Why?
Carol:	I don't want him to feel frustrated.
Dean:	Okay. But in the earlier example, you didn't want to apologize to him. What's different now?
Carol:	Because I don't feel attacked; this is his feeling.
Dean:	Okay. So, what do you say to Bob now?
Carol:	I apologize, Bob.
Dean:	Do you want to know more about why he is frustrated?
Carol:	Yeah.
Dean:	Well, ask him.
Carol:	Why do you feel that way?

Dean:	Stop right there. Bob, do you feel attacked by what she just said?
Bob:	No.
Dean:	Now before you answer her, stop a moment and pay attention to what you are feeling.
Bob:	I feel a gentleness and a kindness coming from her.
Dean:	Okay. What are you feeling inside *you?*
Bob:	I feel more at ease. And I want to ask her if there were any important messages that I should know about.
Dean:	Okay. Now, Carol asked why you feel frustrated.
Bob:	Carol, the reason I was frustrated is because I like to hear my messages firsthand so I can hear the voice of the person.
Dean:	Carol, are you feeling attacked or judged?
Carol:	Not at all. I want to cooperate with him.
Dean:	When you are in a loving relationship, your partner probably likes to please you and to help you. That is one reason why you are together. As soon as your partner feels attacked or judged, even if he

or she otherwise would do just about anything for you, you may find them doing just the opposite of what you want. A judgment from a loved one often resonates with our own inner dialogue when we are critical of ourselves. When we don't push those buttons, it is much easier for your partner to give you what you want. Now, Carol feels free to say, "Well, of course, I'll help you. I won't get your messages. You get your messages," instead of feeling unappreciated, unloved, and misunderstood. It all stems back from feeling judged or criticized. Thank you both very much. I really appreciate it.

Here is another example, this time from a more life-and-death disagreement:

[*Ted and Alice volunteer.*]

Ted: Well, I guess I can start. The biggest argument we've had recently was when I was in the hospital in Des Moines recently after an angioplasty.

Alice: We were on vacation, and we were

riding our bikes through Iowa. It was 108 degrees. Ted was cooking for seventy-five people every night after the bike ride, and there was a lot of stress between us — I didn't want to be around him. I knew something was going to give. One day he told me that he didn't feel very good, so we went to the hospital near the campgrounds. They took us by ambulance to a hospital in Des Moines. The cardiologist said, "You're pretty lucky you made it here."

I'm standing by his bed, looking at him after the nurses left, and I said, "It's almost 110 degrees out there. Wasn't this dumb? You know, it was really stupid that we went on this long bike ride in the heat, and then you had to cook and do all this other stuff. I told you we shouldn't have gone. It almost cost your life. You should have thought about it before you put us in this predicament." Then I told him all the things that we'd already been through that he already knew that we had already been through. And then we had to call the family.

Ted: They all called me stupid, too.

Alice: What did you say in return?

Ted: I became very defensive. I told her, "I don't think I did anything wrong." I tried to prove to her that the things that I was doing were proper and that any other normal person would be doing the things that I was doing.

Dean: Ted, what did you feel when she said that?

Ted: Well, I felt criticized. My next statement right back to her was, "*You're* crazy, and if you would stop nagging, I wouldn't be here. My stress all comes from you! I wouldn't be in the hospital if I didn't have stress from you."

Dean: Alice, how did you feel when he said that?

Alice: Well, he's always said, "You are my stress." And then after I think about it, I think, "Well, maybe you're right. I am your stress." But then, I have to go with the way that I think is right.

Dean: We're just reenacting what happened, but I can still feel the tension. Do you feel closer to each other than before we started this?

Ted: By all means, no.

Dean: Now, can you remember a time when you felt really close and intimate?

Ted: Oh, yes. Many times.

Dean: Imagine one of those times, how good it felt.

Ted: Oh, a typical one would be like when one of our kids got married.

Dean: How did you feel then?

Ted: Wonderful.

Dean: How did you feel then, Alice?

Alice: Great!

Dean: In those moments when you feel intimate, does that feel good?

Alice: Yes.

Dean: How did you feel in the hospital?

Ted: Horrible!

Dean: If we can remember how good it feels to feel intimate, which is usually why we get into relationships in the first place, and how bad it feels when we feel isolated, then the pain can be a powerful motivator of saying, "Maybe we can go about it in a different way." When you said, "I told you so" and, "That was really stupid," then Ted felt judged and attacked back by saying, "You're crazy" and, "I wouldn't be in the hospital if I didn't have stress from you." Those are thoughts, judgments, and criticisms. Alice, what were you feelings when you were standing by his bedside?

Alice: Well, I'm sad, and I am very frustrated because it's a predicament that I can't fix. I was feeling helpless.

Dean: And what else? Were you scared?

Alice: Yes, very scared.

Dean: What were you scared of?

Alice: Scared of not knowing what is happening or what will happen.

Dean: What is the worst that might happen?

Alice: That he could die.

Dean: Now, I want you to just tell him these feelings that you just said you're having.

Alice: Ted, I feel sad, and I feel helpless, and I feel scared that you are going to die and I don't want you to die.

Dean: Why?

Alice: Because I need you. Your whole family needs you. I'll kill you if you die!

Audience: [*Laughter*]

Dean: Ted, the last comment notwithstanding, how do you feel when she says that?

Ted: I can accept it better. It's not like I'm being downgraded or . . .

Dean: Those are thoughts. How do you feel?

Ted: Oh, I feel wonderful. It's soothing to hear that.

Dean: Tell Alice how you feel.

Ted: When you say that to me like that, I understand you more, I feel closer to you. I can accept what you are saying. I feel much better.

Alice: I also feel much happier and closer to Ted.

Dean: And to whatever degree these feelings of closeness affect our survival, you are enhancing the chance of him making a better recovery at the same time. Whatever time you have together, you are not going to waste it feeling more lonely and isolated from each other.

Alice: I feel thankful.

Dean: Thank you very much.

This is an exercise, but these techniques are very powerful in real life. When you are in the heat of it and somebody says something that gets you upset and you have strong emotions, how do you stop and remember that you have different choices other than attacking or withdrawing?

You might say, "Wait a minute. I don't want you to talk to me that way. I am feeling frustrated. I feel attacked. I feel judged. I don't like this. Why don't we take a time-out? Let's come back and discuss this when we are both calmer." There are several different strategies that you can use once you understand the basic principles.

One of the favorite mantras of my colleague and close friend Dr. Jim Billings is, "Remember what you need to remember when you need to remember it." The way you remember is by practicing.

Mahatma Gandhi used to say "Ram," the name of a Hindu god, over and over. When asked, "Why do you do that?" he replied, "I believe that if you say God's name when you die, then you go to heaven. Since I never know when that moment will come, I say it all the time." According to bystanders, his last word when he was assassinated was "Ram," because that is what he was saying most of the time anyway. Whether or not this story is true, if you practice something throughout your daily life, then you are able to draw on it when you most need it.

Of course, there are some people with whom you may not want to be close. There is an old story about a saint who rescues a scorpion that is drowning in the river. He pulls it out of the river and saves the scorpion, which stings him in return. He asks, "Why did you do that? I just saved your life!" The scorpion replied, "I am a scorpion; what do you expect? It's my nature."

Even so, I believe the possibility of transformation is there for most people. In the meantime, sometimes it is appropriate and healthy to have a wall around your heart. It's not always a good idea for you to be defenseless. It may not be safe to do that. But at least we want to be able to let down our walls at home.

It takes a lot of energy to maintain that wall, to hold in and hold back our thoughts and feelings. Over time, this can lead to great suffering and illness. If you can't open up with your own wife or loved ones, then you have a problem. That doesn't mean you should always keep your heart open to everyone, because there are some mean people out there. At the same time, if you routinely come into contact with a difficult person, you may want to at least give him or her a chance to change. I find that if I can use good communication skills on my end, it often makes it easier for them to change — but not always. If it doesn't happen, then I might say, "Fine, you stay in your corner; I will stay in mine."

As a side note, I spoke at the National Governors' Association annual meeting in 1997 to the fifty state governors and their spouses. I went through a similar communication skills exercise with them. When I began the exercise by saying, "I think you are wrong! And I think you're a jerk! How does that feel?" they replied, "Familiar . . ."

Group Support

Why is group support, which I discussed in chapter 2, so powerful? It provides a safe place for people consciously to choose to let down their emotional defenses and barriers in order to practice expressing their emotions and opening their hearts to each other. When people open their hearts to each other, healing often happens.[1]

More precisely, *a support group helps heal isolation, alienation, and loneliness.* When this happens, physical healing often follows, from the inside out. Healing is a process of becoming whole. If we define healing as avoiding death, then sooner or later we're going to fail 100 percent of the time. As I wrote in chapter 1, we may heal our suffering even when curing the physical disease is not possible, although often both healing and curing may transpire.

Healing means that you are more at ease, more at peace, that you have a sense of connection and connectedness and a sense of being more in touch with your soul's purpose. Many people find their values change when they are diagnosed with a life-threatening illness. Suddenly, accomplishment, money, power, fame, and fortune are not nearly as important to them as being with people for whom they care, whom they love, and by whom they feel nurtured and loved.

There are many kinds of support groups. Many focus on coping with a particular disease, addiction, or problem: Alcoholics Anonymous, Mended Hearts, and so on. Other groups focus on psychopathology: depression, schizophrenia, and other disorders. The group support in our research is different. Our focus is to create an intentional community of people who are committed to healing loneliness and isolation.

I believe that whatever else is going on in these other groups, a common denominator that may well be responsible for much of their success is the feeling of connection and community shared by group members even when this feeling is a by-product of the group experience rather than an actual goal.

Group support has been part of my research since my first study in 1977. The original purpose of the group was to help people stay on the *other* parts of the program — how to follow the diet, exercise, practice yoga, and so on. I began to learn that what these research participants needed most was a place where they could talk openly with each other. The group was not just a way to help people adhere to the other parts of the program. I discovered that the group experience *was* perhaps the most important component of the intervention.

At first, I would tend to problem-solve during the group sessions. These groups often turned into "ask the doctor," and I found myself spending much of the time answering questions, offering advice, and trying to fix whatever was wrong.

Later, Dr. Billings helped me to understand that even when we couldn't fix the external problem — for example, the teenage son at home addicted to heroin, the stress at work — we could begin to heal the loneliness and isolation. Along the way, the group participants began to see that feeling loved and supported made the other problems seem more manageable and tolerable even when they couldn't be solved. I learned to refrain from giving advice and, instead, to listen with empathy and to encourage the group members to express their feelings rather than their questions. There were other opportunities in different settings for questions and answers.

When someone feels heard and understood, even when the son is still on heroin, the sense of intimacy grows so much that the suffering is more tolerable. Feeling supported and intimate allows someone to feel good enough to address some of the core issues of a problem — in this case, what may have contributed to his son's addiction. We can't always fix the problems out there, but at least we can begin to heal our own sense of separation, isolation, and loneliness.

In a real and intentional way, we are trying to recreate something that has been part of the human experience until recently — a place where other people know you, warts and all, and they are still there. They accept you as you are, and they *love* you as you are, even when they don't necessarily *like* everything about you.

Many people rarely, if ever, have experienced how good it feels to be accepted in this way. If you can't really open your heart to someone, if you can't really show all of yourself — not just what you consider the good stuff — then you are limiting how intimate you can be. The fear is often, "If you really knew me, you wouldn't want to be with me, so I have to create a façade of who I want you to *think* I am that is more lovable and acceptable than who I *really* am."

When people hide their fears behind a mask, they tend to feel even more lonely, no matter what happens. If they don't receive love and respect, then they lose. Even if they do feel loved and respected, they often can't enjoy it because they know it's only for part of them. One patient told me, "They don't love *me*, they love this *image* of me. If they *really* knew what I was like, if they knew my dark side, then they'd be out of here."

They may become vigilant to hide those parts that they think are unlovable, which can be enormously stressful. Worse, they may think they're alone in feeling this way — because, by definition, they have few people with whom to talk openly. With constant vigilance comes chronic stress and often enormous suffering.

Part of what makes our support groups so powerful is that people begin to realize that they are not alone. We try to create a safe environment that gives them permission to talk about what they are really feeling — "Here's what's really going on in my life" — and to encourage people to listen with empathy and compassion, without judging them, rejecting them, abandoning them, or trying to fix them.

Part of the value of a stable community, neighborhood, and extended family is that people know you. They know your secrets. Gossip is society's way of spreading everyone's secrets around a neighborhood. *You* know that *they* know, and *they* know that *you* know that *they* know — and they are still there for you. They are still your neighbors, and they still talk to you. It's a great relief. As Oscar Wilde wrote in *The Picture of Dorian Gray* in 1891, "There is only one thing in the world worse than being talked about, and that is not being talked about."

In our groups, people begin to see each other on a soul level, through loving eyes rather than in a judgmental way. At first, though, people see the differences. They see all the ways in which we categorize people — differences in age, race, religion, gender, sexual preference, socioeconomic status, demographics, where they went to school, what kind of car they drive, what kind of clothes they wear — all of the differences we can use to separate each other by feeling better than or less than somebody else.

At the beginning of the first group, a common feeling is, "What have I gotten myself into? I don't think I even like some of these people. I can't imagine opening up to them." As the author Parker Palmer has noted, community is the place where the person you least want to be with shows up. Yet this is precisely what makes the experience so healing: finding out how much we have in common with the people we avoid or dislike.

Over time, our group participants begin to talk about their feelings. They really begin to trust each other. They begin to open up and open their hearts to each other. They begin to talk about what is real for them. They realize that while the external forms and categorizations may differ, on a soul level we have similar feelings, desires, fears, hopes, wishes, and dreams.

The essence of compassion — which is the essence of healing — is to realize that we are not so different from each other in the experience of being human. We all want to be happy and to avoid suffering. At its best, the group is a spiritual experience: seeing, feeling, and understanding the interconnectedness rather than only the differences. This interconnectedness can be experienced in direct ways through meditation and prayer, but the experience of this *human* dimension of our interconnectedness can be quite profound and wonderful. Although I have led hundreds of groups, it is always magic to me to watch this process unfold. As Henry Wadsworth Longfellow wrote, "If we could read the secret history of our enemies, we should find in each man's life sorrow and suffering enough to disarm all hostility."

People who come to our weeklong retreats are often familiar with my books and understand the purpose of the groups. They are ready to do this work. Even so, we find it extraordinary to watch a group of people who are total strangers to each other make a commitment to the group process and begin opening their hearts to each other. Often, by the end of the first day, they are sharing stories and secrets with each other that their own families and friends might not know.

In some respects, it is easier to open up with total strangers, because there is no history of wounding, fighting, and arguing with them. I often find this to be true on airplanes, where people who are total strangers sitting next to me often begin disclosing intimate details of their lives as we fly across the country.

In our support groups, there is a commitment to the common purpose of opening up. We use the communication skills I described in the preceding section:

- Identify what you are feeling.
- Disclose what you are feeling.
- Listen carefully to what the other person is feeling.
- Acknowledge the other person's feelings with empathy, caring, and compassion.

When people begin to experience how good it feels to open in this way, they develop the motivation and the skills to begin applying these approaches in their own lives and relationships.

We encourage people to reveal who they really are and what they are really feeling. In addition to focusing on how people communicate feelings, we also encourage people to *listen actively and empathically.* The experience of feeling heard by another person is healing; equally beneficial is the experience of listening fully to another person and to his or her experiences.

When a person has finished talking, we ask members of the group to relate whatever feelings were evoked in them by the other person. This process — empathy — is the experience of feelings that arise in you in response to emotions communicated by another. If the members of a group are experiencing empathy for what a person has just communicated, then everyone in the group is connected in that moment by that common experience.

Sharing feelings rather than attacking or criticizing makes it easier for others to listen; listening leads to empathy; empathy leads to compassion; compassion increases intimacy; intimacy is healing.

We ask everyone to resist the natural inclination to give advice on how to solve the problem (unless someone specifically asks for it) and, instead, to focus on feeling and expressing his or her own emotions and experiences. Remember: The problem we are trying to solve is a lack of intimacy, not the kid on drugs or the boss at work. The lack of intimacy can be solved even when the other problems cannot.

This process takes courage and practice. It is unfamiliar to many people precisely because the experience of intimacy is so rare and precious in our culture. Although many of our research participants were initially skeptical — and sometimes even hostile — to the group support process, most later said that they found the group support to be the most meaningful, helpful, and powerful part of their experience.

As we have seen, increasing scientific evidence documents the healing benefits of opening your heart. Many studies have shown that self-disclosure — that is, talking or even writing about your feelings to others — improves physical health, enhances immune function, reduces cardiovascular reactivity, decreases absentee rates, and may even prolong life.

Much of this important work has been conducted by James Pennebaker and his colleagues.[2-6] While disclosure of *facts* is helpful, disclosure of *feelings* is much more powerful.[7] The researchers also found that disclosure of traumatic or painful experiences had a more powerful benefit on health and healing than talking or writing about superficial events, even if in the short run the person felt worse. They found that the greater the degree of disclosure, the more benefits they measured. These benefits persisted over time. The benefits were particularly striking in those who talked about upsetting or traumatic experiences they had not previously discussed with others in detail. According to Dr. Pennebaker,

My own belief is that the most interesting and perhaps potent benefit of social support is in providing an outlet for people to talk about their thoughts and feelings. In large surveys with corporate employees as well as college students, for example, we find the same thing that other social-support researchers have shown: The more friends you have, the healthier you are. However, this effect is due, almost exclusively, to the degree which you have talked with your friends about any traumas that you have suffered.

But here's the kicker. If you have had a trauma that you have not talked about with anyone, the number of friends you have is unrelated to your health. Social support only protects your health if you use it wisely. That is, if you have suffered a major upheaval in your life, talk to your friends about it. Merely having friends is not enough.[8]

You may want to begin by writing your thoughts and feelings in a journal or diary. You can be completely honest and open because you're safe; no one will judge, abandon, or criticize you. Problems that might seem disturbing or even overwhelming often begin to seem more manageable when you see them on paper. Although writing in a journal does not heal the isolation between you and others, it can help you articulate your feelings and thus be a powerful means of reintegrating and healing the distance between you and your own feelings.

If you want to create your own group, I suggest that you include only those people who share the goal of healing isolation and are willing to make a commitment to attend regularly. You may find the communication skills described here to be very helpful. The point of the group is to create a safe environment for people to be honest and self-disclosing. Even one person who is hostile to this process or who comes only sporadically tends to make everyone else feel unsafe. Each group member might decide to pay part of the cost of a trained group leader, or you may choose to do it on your own.

Don't worry too much about whether or not you are doing it "right"; after all, the goal is to recreate and regain a lost sense of extended family and community that has been with us for hundreds of thousands of years. The goal is to apply these skills and principles that you practice in the group to enhance intimacy in the relationships that are the most important to you: with your spouse or significant other, with your family, with your friends, with your colleagues, with your community.

Confession, Forgiveness, and Redemption

The group support process of self-disclosure is somewhat related to the process of confession, forgiveness, and redemption that is part of most religious and spiritual traditions. These help us to open our hearts. For example, the following passage is from a prayer book used on Yom Kippur, the Jewish Day of Atonement: "A new heart will I give you, a new spirit put within you. I will remove the heart of stone from your flesh, and give you a heart that feels."[9]

The reasons and procedures may differ from one religion to another, but the underlying principle is the same. On the Day of Atonement, for example, Jews confess as a group to avoid any particular member feeling stigmatized. In Judaism, as in most religions, confessing to God does not absolve a person from the need to confess, ask pardon, and make restitution to a person whom he or she may have wronged. Forgiving the abuser and his or her ignorance does not condone the abuse.

During the crucifixion, Jesus demonstrated by example a profound act of compassion and forgiveness while nailed to the cross: "Father, forgive them; for they know not what they do."[10] Some branches of Christianity encourage followers to confess their perceived shortcomings to their priests or ministers, others in the presence of the congregation, others in prayer or to oneself. Buddhism, Hinduism, Islam, Native American religions, and others have similar rituals and practices involving confession, forgiveness, and redemption. The very reason that most cultures have developed a way for people to disclose and share their deepest and often darkest feelings is because the healing benefits are so strong. The issue I am discussing here is not God's judgment, but our own.

When you can share your darkest secrets and mistakes with another person who listens without judgment, it is like shining a light in the darkness. A powerful social bond of intimacy is forged with the listener. Equally important, you reintegrate those parts of yourself that may have been split off because they seemed the most painful and the least lovable. In short, you become more intimate with the deepest parts of yourself.

When someone else can have compassion, forgiveness, and acceptance of those dark parts of ourselves that seem so unlovable, it makes it easier for us to accept those parts within us. When we can do this, we are less likely to project our darkness onto others and hate them. If we don't acknowledge our anger, for example, we are more prone to violence. Instead, as we have more compassion for our own weaknesses and foibles, it becomes easier to feel more empathy and forgiveness for the ignorance and darkness that we experience in others. This experience is healing for the one asking for forgiveness as well as for the other who is offering it.

Sometimes I find it helpful to remind myself that we are all in different stages of our growth and evolution. Someone who does not yet have a great capacity for intimacy or forgiveness now may develop it later. Even if the other person is not ready to accept our forgiveness — "whose heart cannot yet see," in the words of the Vietnamese meditation master Thich Nhat Hanh — forgiveness helps to free *us* in the meantime.

Even in secular culture, celebrities and politicians are finding that confession allows the American public to forgive a multitude of unwise choices. The actor Hugh Grant, for example, was caught with a prostitute in his car in Los Angeles. In what has now become a familiar American ritual, he appeared soon thereafter on Jay Leno's television show expressing remorse and self-deprecation. In that moment, viewers were transformed into priests or close friends. Indeed, public opinion polls later showed that the actor's popularity became higher than it had been before the incident with the prostitute occurred.

There is a dark side to self-disclosure, like all powerful forces. Many cults and street gangs require members to disclose their secrets as a way of creating strong bonds to the organization. Political movements such as the Cultural Revolution in China often required jailed political dissidents to sign statements or appear on television "confessing" their remorse and publicly criticizing their own views. Some American prisoners of war during the Vietnam War and those held hostage in Iran during the 1980s had similar experiences.

At its best, though, self-disclosure and forgiveness are powerful forces for healing the loneliness and isolation that often separate us from each other and from parts of ourselves that we have kept hidden in darkness for too long.

There are many examples of forgiveness meditations. Some are simple, others are more elaborate. Rather than telling you how

I think you should forgive, I believe it is more meaningful for you to search your own heart and do what feels authentic and comfortable. For example, you can find an extended forgiveness meditation in the book *Embracing the Beloved*, by Stephen and Ondrea Levine.

It bears repeating: Forgiveness does not condone or excuse someone from their actions in hurting you; rather, it helps empower and free you from the pain of chronic anger, separation, and isolation.

You may want to begin by finding a comfortable place, closing your eyes, and bringing to mind someone who hurt you, knowingly or unknowingly. Notice how your body feels and how your mind feels when you have a mental image of them doing what was hurtful to you. You may feel disturbed, angry, upset, or in pain. These feelings may get called up in your body and mind whenever you think of this person; thus, it may be in your own best interest to let go of what happened. When you think of this person with anger, it does not affect him or her, but it may be causing real problems for *you*. In whatever way feels appropriate and comfortable for you, consider letting go of your anger and, with it, your pain: "I forgive you." I sometimes find it helpful to think of the person as ignorant rather than malicious.

You may then want to extend that same compassion to yourself. Many people find it harder to forgive themselves than to forgive someone else. Again, close your eyes and bring to mind an incident in which you did something hurtful to someone else that you regret. Notice how your body feels and how your mind feels when you have a mental image of yourself doing what was hurtful to the other person. You may feel disturbed, angry, upset, or in pain. These feelings may get called up in your body and mind whenever you think of this incident; thus, it may be in your own best interest to let go of what happened. In whatever way feels appropriate and comfortable for you, consider letting go of your anger toward yourself and, with it, your pain. "I forgive you."

Compassion, Altruism, and Service

Do you want to be Mother Teresa or Donald Trump? Do you choose to help only yourself *or* do you choose to help others?

Trick question. Fortunately you don't have to choose.

When you help others, you also help yourself. Seen from that perspective, helping others — being unselfish — is the most "selfish" of all activities, for that is what helps to free us from our loneliness and isolation and suffering.

Compassion, altruism, and service — like confession, forgiveness, and redemption — are part of almost all religious and spiritual traditions as well as many secular ones. We are hardwired to help each other. This has helped us survive as a species for the past several hundred thousand years.

In the Tecumseh Community Health Study described in chapter 2, for example, almost three thousand men and women were studied for nine to twelve years. After adjustments for age and a variety of risk factors for mortality, men reporting higher levels of social relationships and activities were significantly less likely to die during the follow-up period. Some social activities were more protective than others. The investigators found that activities involving regular volunteer work were among the most powerful predictors of reduced mortality rates. Those who volunteered to help others at least once a week were two and a half times less likely to die during the study as those who never volunteered. In other words, *those who helped others lived longer themselves.*[11]

In another study, researchers at Cornell University followed 427 married women with children for thirty years beginning in

1956. When they began the study, the researchers hypothesized that housewives with more children would be under greater stress with fewer options and thus would be more likely to die prematurely.

They were surprised to find that *women who were members of volunteer organizations lived longer.* Other factors such as number of children, whether or not a woman worked in an office or as a housewife, education, social class, and so on did not affect longevity. Specifically, 52 percent of women who did not belong to a volunteer organization at the beginning of the study were found to have experienced a major illness thirty years later compared with only 36 percent of women who had belonged to a volunteer organization.[12]

Just as chronic stress can suppress your immune function, altruism, love, and compassion may enhance it. In chapter 2, I described a study of students at Harvard who were asked to watch a documentary movie about Mother Teresa's service to the sick and dying poor of Calcutta's worst slums. Another group of students watched a more neutral film. On average those who watched the movie about Mother Teresa showed a significant increase in protective antibodies whereas those who watched the neutral film did not.[13] In other words, just watching a film of someone embodying altruism improved immune function.

Studies of volunteers have shown that not only do they tend to live longer, but also they often feel better, sometimes reporting a sudden burst of endorphins similar to a "runner's high" while helping others. This good feeling that comes from helping others is a subset of a larger context: *Anything that helps us freely choose to transcend the boundaries of separateness is joyful.* When you volunteer, you have a choice. When you are pressured or coerced to meet someone else's needs, the joy of helping and the health benefits are compromised or even counterproductive.

At its best, making love is an ecstatic experience when two lovers merge as one, opening their hearts to each other and melting the boundaries that separate them. After my first sexual experience as a teenager, however, I remember thinking, "Is that it? That's all?" There was a brief physiological release but hardly an ecstatic experience. Only much later in life, when I learned to make love with an open heart, did I begin to understand how joyful it could be. There is a growing interest in tantra and other approaches that help couples learn to combine sexuality and spirituality.

The ecstasy that comes from melting the boundaries between self and other is also part of most religious and spiritual traditions. While there are many pathways to experiencing God or the Self, praying with an open heart is one of the most powerful and joyful. Someone might choose to live a celibate life as a monk or a nun or a swami or a priest out of repression or fear of one's sexual impulses, but at its highest form they might renounce worldly relationships because the feelings of ecstasy and freedom that come from merging with God, with the Self, are so much more powerful even than merging with one's beloved mate. Indeed, in this sacred tradition God is often referred to as the Beloved. As I wrote in the previous chapter, there is no point in giving up something you enjoy unless what you get back is even better. In this tradition, people believe they are giving up a worldly life for the direct experience of God — a good trade-off.

Seen from the highest perspective, we see others as incarnations of God, of the Self, *as* our self. On a more human level, Dr. James Lynch writes, "The mandate to 'Love your neighbor as you love yourself' is not just a moral mandate. It's a physiological mandate. Caring is biological. One thing you get from caring for others is you're not lonely. And the more connected you are to life, the healthier you are."[14]

Thus, the reason altruism may be healing for both the giver and the recipient is that giving to others with an open heart helps heal the isolation that appears to separate us from each other. While the forms and rituals of the various religious and spiritual traditions vary, underneath these differences is a common view: On one level, we are separate from everyone and everything, the self with a small "s." You are your self, and I am my self. On another level, though, we are part of something larger that connects us all — the universal Self, by any other name: God, Buddha, Spirit, Allah, whatever.

Even to give a name is to limit it. When God was revealed to Moses, he asked, "When I tell the people that the God of their fathers has sent me, they will ask his name. What shall I tell them?" And God said, "*I am what I am.* Tell them *I am* has sent you."[15]

As I wrote in the previous chapter, the vision of unity consciousness and oneness is found in virtually all cultures and all religions. God or the Self is described as omniscient, omnipresent, and omnipotent. As described in the Old Testament, "The Lord is One." If God is everywhere, omnipresent,

One, then we are not separate from God.

What we experience as different names and forms is God or the Self in varying disguises, manifesting in different ways. All divisions are man-made. The word *yoga* is Sanskrit for "union." A central precept in Hinduism is "Thou art that. . . . The universe is nothing but Brahman."[16] According to Jesus, "The kingdom of God is within you."[17] Buddha taught, "You are all Buddhas. There is nothing that you need to achieve. Just open your eyes."[18] The Arabian prophet Muhammad, founder of Islam, wrote, "Wherever you turn is God's face. . . . Whoever knows himself knows God."[19] Albert Einstein, the greatest scientist of the twentieth century, wrote, "The true value of a human being can be found in the degree to which he has attained liberation from the [separate] self."[20]

The writer Aldous Huxley called this the "perennial philosophy."[21] This vision is at the heart of compassion. From this perspective, "Love your neighbor as your Self" is a statement of fact, of what is, rather than a commandment.[22] For those who may not yet realize this truth, this commandment is also a signpost pointing the way to a path that can help them experience the Self. As written in the *Upanishads* over 2,500 years ago (translated by the poet W. B. Yeats and others):

> That is perfect. This is perfect. Perfect comes from perfect. Take perfect from perfect, the remainder is perfect.
>
> May peace and peace and peace be everywhere.
>
> The Self is everywhere, without a body, without a shape, whole, pure, wise, all knowing, far shining, self-depending, all transcending; in the eternal procession assigning to every period its proper duty.[23]

This experience is sometimes described as Oneness or at other times as complete emptiness, void; more precisely, as both. This paradox — everything and nothing — is at the heart of the transcendent experience, "an immediate, nondual insight that transcends conceptualization,"[24] for it is our concepts of how we *think* things are that often keep us from seeing and experiencing how they *really* are.

By analogy, Swami Satchidananda describes the one light in a movie projector manifesting as an entire universe of people, places, and dramas on the movie screen. When we can maintain this double vision — seeing the different names and forms while remembering it's just a movie and seeing the one light behind the many images — then we can more fully enjoy the movie without getting lost in it, without forgetting who we really are.

Although this experience of Oneness lies beyond the intellect, it can be directly experienced. Compassion naturally flows when the divisions that separate us from each other begin to fade.

Compassion helps to free us from anger. Anger itself is often a manifestation of the misperception that we are separate and only separate.

Shantideva was an Indian scholar who lived in the eighth century. His classic work, *The Way of the Bodhisattva*, describes in approximately eight hundred verses the path of the bodhisattva: those who vow to work for the enlightenment of all beings. It describes how compassion and concern for others is at the center of all spiritual practices and wisdom:

All the joy the world contains
Has come through wishing happiness for
   others.
All the misery the world contains
Has come through wanting pleasure for
   oneself [at the expense of others].[25]

To cultivate compassion, Shantideva provides a detailed meditation that involves seeing yourself through your opponent's eyes. Imagine that you are looking back at yourself through the other person's eyes. First, see yourself in an inferior position (while feeling envy for yourself); then, as an equal (while feeling rivalry and competitiveness); then in a superior position (while feeling pride and condescension toward yourself). Experience what it feels like to be on the receiving end of your own behavior.

When you can do this — which is a form of visualization — then you gain a greater appreciation of why others feel the way they do and how you appear in their eyes. In short, you gain greater compassion and empathy. This is more than just sympathy for the plight of others. When we can transcend the distinction between ourselves and others, then the suffering of others becomes as real to us as our own.

This attitude is embodied in the lecture given by the Dalai Lama when he was awarded the Nobel Peace Prize in 1989. He described his feelings about the Chinese who have occupied Tibet during the past forty years:

I speak not with a feeling of anger or

hatred towards those who are responsible for the immense suffering of our people and the destruction of our land, homes, and culture. They, too, are human beings who struggle to find happiness and deserve our compassion. I speak to inform you of the sad situation in my country today and of the aspirations of my people, because in our struggle for freedom, truth is the only weapon we possess.

The realization that we are all basically the same human beings, who seek happiness and try to avoid suffering, is very helpful in developing a sense of brotherhood and sisterhood — a warm feeling of love and compassion for others. This, in turn, is essential if we are to survive in this ever-shrinking world we live in. For if we each selfishly pursue only what we believe to be in our own interest, without caring about the needs of others, we may end up harming not only others but also ourselves. . . .

Peace, for example, starts within each one of us. Then we have inner peace, we can be at peace with those around us. When our community is in a state of peace, it can share that peace with neighboring communities and so on. When we feel love and kindness towards others, it not only makes others feel loved and cared for but it helps us also to develop inner happiness and peace.

This level of compassion is beyond the capacity of what I and most other people can do at this stage in our spiritual development. Imagine: Your country has been overrun by invaders, your homes and temples destroyed, many thousands of people killed and tortured, and you are living in exile — and you respond not with hatred but with compassion.

While many are inspired by such feats of compassion, others may be intimidated, since this is so far removed from the capacity and daily experience of most people. It is important to remember that even the smallest acts of compassion — for yourself and for others — have benefits. The more we experience these benefits, the more encouraged we become to do even more. Our emotional and spiritual hearts, like the muscle of our physical heart, grow stronger with practice. Do what you can comfortably, and leave the rest. In a real sense, our enemies are our teachers because they provide us the opportunity to practice compassion. After all, it's easy to love our friends, or, as Oscar Wilde once said, "It's not the perfect but the imperfect that is in need of our love." Truth is truth; Jesus said, "Love your enemies, do good to those who hate you, bless those who curse you, and pray for those who mistreat you."[26]

In the name of compassion, people sometimes allow themselves to be abused. Avoid giving more than feels comfortable to you. Give when it comes from a genuine place in your heart, for the sake of giving, not out of guilt or fear or because someone else thinks it's what you *should* be doing. Avoid using the gratitude of others as a means of propping up a wounded self-image. Remember, you can only say yes to giving freely when you can also choose to say no.

Psychotherapy

Psychotherapy can be a very helpful complement to spiritual practices. When I was nineteen and severely depressed, I needed to see a therapist just to become stable enough to function. At the same time, the deeper answers I was seeking were not to be found in Western schools of psychiatry or psychology; I benefited from both psychotherapy and spiritual practices and found useful tools in each for learning to live more skillfully and more joyfully.

Some people believe that meditation, prayer, and related spiritual practices can heal all problems, but I am not one of them. Many unresolved issues having to do with family, self-esteem, boundaries, developmental issues, grief, intimacy, childhood abuse, addictions, neuroses, and so on are best addressed by a skilled psychotherapist.

There are two basic approaches to psychotherapy: supportive and insight-oriented. Supportive therapy helps you get through the day. Medications, especially antidepressants, are often prescribed. Though supportive therapy can be helpful in making it through a crisis, insight-oriented therapy helps you gain more awareness of the underlying patterns and causes that led to the problems. There are many different schools and approaches in both supportive and insight-oriented therapy. Unfortunately, there is a growing trend for insurance companies to reimburse short-term, drug-based supportive therapy rather than longer-term insight-oriented approaches.

Choose carefully if you decide to explore psychotherapy. A superb therapist — like an outstanding spiritual teacher or, for that matter, an excellent golf instructor — is hard to find but it is worth the effort. Look for a therapist who has good boundaries, a place where you can feel safe enough to delve into issues and wounds that are often by nature painful to explore. Interview several; afterwards, meditate on whether or not the person seems right for you. Your heart will know; if you ask, and if you listen, it may tell you. Who the therapist is — what he or she embodies — is often more important than any particular technique or training.

At best, spiritual practices and psychotherapy complement one another. Meditation, for example, may increase your awareness of disturbing feelings or ideas; a good therapist can help you understand the developmental and emotional issues that may be underlying those thoughts and feelings. Opening up and sharing secrets with a therapist provides both emotional and spiritual benefits of self-disclosure and feeling heard that I described earlier in this chapter, especially if he or she can provide insight without judgment.

Spiritual practices and psychotherapy are particularly valuable in exploring issues related to intimacy. For example, therapy can help define boundaries and a well-developed separate sense of self; spiritual practices can help expand that awareness from the separate self to the universal Self. As we have discussed, one must first have a well-defined separate self in order to transcend it. Recognizing only our separateness leads to loneliness and suffering; recognizing only our Oneness makes it difficult to function in the world. Combining psychotherapy and spiritual practices can help maintain a vision of both the diversity and unity of life.

There is still an unfortunate belief among many people that psychotherapy is only for those who are crazy or severely disturbed. In politics, for example, there is a perceived stigma of having been to a psychotherapist even though this is one arena where it may be most needed. I hope for a time when someone running for elected office can say, "Yes, I have worked hard on myself in psychotherapy, and this makes me a more qualified candidate."

When I began seeing a therapist at age nineteen, he said, "Tell me about your mother and father." "Well, *that's* an original question from a therapist," I thought derisively. I learned that those relationships really do matter — not to blame but to understand, so that we can be free to consider new choices.

In chapter 2, I described two studies of people who reported not feeling close to one or both parents when they were students at

Harvard and at Johns Hopkins in the 1940s and 1950s. Thirty-five to fifty years later, they were much more likely to have developed serious illnesses and to have died prematurely in midlife.

Why should how we relate to our parents earlier in life affect our health and survival decades later? An important reason why early family relationships are so predictive of later illness is that *these patterns of relating do not change very much in most people over time.* Whether or not it was safe for you to be open and intimate in your family while growing up may determine to a large degree how safe it feels for you to be in an intimate relationship now. This view of the world — is it safe to open my heart and make myself vulnerable? — is molded during early years of development.

These patterns of relating do not change very much in most people over time because our culture does not often encourage us to examine these issues. When you understand how addressing early developmental issues can increase your capacity for intimacy and joy now, then you may become more motivated to consider working with a good therapist where you can practice being vulnerable and emotionally intimate in a safe environment so that you can then apply these skills outside the therapist's office. When we understand how powerfully love and intimacy affect not only the quality and joy in our lives but also our very survival, then we may become more motivated to explore whatever approaches may be of value — including all of those described in this chapter, and more.

Touching

What is the largest organ in your body? Your skin. We all know that a loving touch feels good, but did you know it can also affect your health and even your survival?

Intimacy is healing. Touching is intimate. Lack of human contact can lead to profound isolation and illness — and even death.

The relationship of touching to health was noted as far back as the thirteenth century. The German emperor Frederick II conducted a horrible experiment to find out what language children would speak if they were raised without hearing anyone talking. He took several newborns away from their parents and gave them to nurses who were forbidden to touch or talk with them. These babies never learned a language because they all died before they could talk. In the year 1248, the historian Salimbene wrote of these babies, "They could not live without petting."[27]

More recently, a study of babies in ten institutions in 1915 found that every baby who was less than two years old had died, even though nutrition and sanitation were adequate. Why? Concern about spreading infectious diseases led to a policy of minimal human contact with the babies, which were touched only infrequently.[28]

A number of studies are now showing the benefits of touch in newborns. At the Touch Research Institute in Miami, premature babies given three loving massages a day for ten days gained weight 47 percent faster and left the hospital six days sooner, saving $10,000 each.[29]

There are hundreds of studies demonstrating the healing value of touch — in cocaine-exposed infants, HIV-exposed infants, infants parented by depressed mothers, and full-term infants without medical problems. Massage has also been found to be useful in treating asthma, autism, back pain, cancer, depression, developmental delays, dermatitis (psoriasis), diabetes, eating disorders (bulimia), heart disease, irregular heart beats, juvenile rheumatoid arthritis, posttraumatic stress disorder, and a variety of other conditions. For example, a study of HIV-positive men found that massage for one month caused a significant increase in both the number and cytotoxicity of natural killer cell activity.[30]

Despite this, we do not touch each other very much in the United States when compared with other parts of the world. Psychologist Sidney Jourard observed and recorded how many times couples in cafés casually touched each other in an hour. The highest rates were in Puerto Rico (180 times per hour) and Paris (110 times per hour). Guess how many times per hour couples touched each other in the United States? Twice! (In London, it was *zero*. They *never* touched.) He also found that French parents and children touched each other three times more frequently than did American parents and children.[31]

Again, awareness is the first step in healing. When we understand the healing power of touching, we can look for ways of increasing our contact with other people while respecting their boundaries. Give someone a pat on the back or a hug when they've done a good job — or even when they haven't. Get a massage or manicure or shampoo. Shake hands when you see a colleague. Hold hands with your beloved — and don't forget to kiss.

Therapeutic touch is a type of massage that also combines the intention of the person to help or heal while in a meditative state. It was pioneered by Dolores Krieger and is increasingly taught and used by nurses and other health practitioners. Therapeutic touch also can be practiced by simply placing your hands near someone rather than on them. The goal is to "rebalance energy" and to stimulate a person's own natural intrinsic healing responses. One of the leading practitioners and researchers of therapeutic touch is Janet Quinn, who described it this way: "Therapeutic touch, at its core, is the offering of unconditional love and compassion. . . . We're here for service. We're here to love other people. . . . The most fundamental longing of the human heart is for union with the Divine."[32, 33]

Commitment

As I wrote earlier, commitment leads to real freedom, in any arena. This is particularly true in relationships of all kinds, for you can only be intimate to the degree that you can be vulnerable. You can only be vulnerable and open your heart to the degree that you feel safe — because if you make yourself vulnerable, you might get hurt. Commitment creates safety and makes intimacy possible.

I said this to my beloved when we made a commitment to each other:

"I commit myself fully to you, for I want this relationship to be as intimate and loving as possible. Our intimacy and love nourish my soul and allow me to experience the most happiness and meaning.

"I am willing to risk making myself more and more vulnerable to you, even though I may get hurt from time to time. I would rather take that risk and have the potential of real intimacy than to wall myself off and have the certainty of being isolated and alone.

"I commit to being completely and totally honest with you, for we can be open and vulnerable with each other only if we can fully trust each other.

"I commit to try to avoid hurting you so that we can create something really sacred. I know there will be times that we may hurt each other, knowingly or unknowingly, but I will do my best not to cause you pain. When that happens, I will ask for your forgiveness and I will offer mine without reservation. When we can make mistakes in a relationship that has become safe and sacred, then knowing we can love and be loved even when we mess up builds even greater trust, makes it feel even safer, and deepens the intimacy.

"I commit to making our relationship the most important priority in our lives. As we spend more time together and learn to trust each other, I hope that our hearts will continue to open more and more and still more to each other."

I do not wish to minimize the difficulties and obstacles to commitment, to romanticize it, or to trivialize it. Commitment is a process, not a goal; with hard work and grace, it deepens over time.

Commitment, like meditation, is focused intentionality. A romantic relationship is only one arena for commitment. You may commit to your child, to your job, to your friends, to your organization, to your country — to anything. We define ourselves by our commitments.

Meditation

Meditation is the practice and process of paying attention and focusing your awareness. When you meditate, a number of desirable things begin to happen — slowly at first, and deepening over time:

First, *when you can focus your awareness, you gain more power.* When you concentrate any form of energy, including mental energy, you gain power. This power may come in many forms. For example, when you focus your mind, you concentrate better. When you concentrate better, you perform better. You can accomplish more, whether in the classroom, in the boardroom, or in the athletic arena. Whatever you do, you do it more effectively when you meditate. It is for this reason that spiritual teachers and texts often caution that one should begin the practice of meditation only in the context of other spiritual practices and disciplines that help develop compassion and wisdom to use properly these increased powers.

Second, *you enjoy your senses more fully.* Although people sometimes view or use meditation as an ascetic experience to *control* their senses, meditation also can *enhance* your senses in ways that are profoundly sensual. Anything that you enjoy — food, sex, music, art, massage, and so on — is greatly enhanced by meditation. When you pay attention to something, it's a lot more enjoyable. Also, you don't need as much of it to get the same degree of pleasure, so you are more likely to enjoy without excess.

When you keep a wall around your heart to armor and protect it from pain, you also diminish your capacity to feel pleasure. When your life is in a continual rush, you may miss exquisite pleasures that exist from moment to moment. Attention spans get shorter. The need for stimulation continually increases just to feel *anything*. The mainstreaming of sadomasochism is one manifestation of this. Meditation increases awareness and sensitivity; as such, it can be an antidote to numbness and distraction and a way of greatly increasing joy and pleasure.

Third, *your mind quiets down and you may experience an inner sense of peace, joy, and well-being*. When I first learned to meditate and began getting glimpses of inner peace, this experience changed my life in ways I described in the previous chapter. It redefined and reframed my experience. Before, I thought peace of mind came from getting and doing; now, I understand that it comes from *being*. It is our true nature to be peaceful until we disturb it.

This is a radically different concept of where our happiness and our well-being come from. In one of life's great paradoxes, not being aware of this truth, we often end up disturbing our inner peace while striving to get or to do what we think will bring that same peace to us.

The idea that peace, joy, and well-being come from outside ourselves is reinforced in so many different ways in our culture. The advertising industry is based on this idea:

"Buy this product and you'll be happy." Advertisers understand the powerful human need for love and intimacy and exploit this desire in order to sell products. When you see an advertisement for a hamburger chain, chances are you won't find someone sitting alone eating by himself or herself. More likely is that you will see a happy family smiling and laughing together. The beer commercial promises, "Proud to be your Bud," your buddy. AT&T implores, "Reach out and touch someone."

As I have written in previous books, so much suffering begins with a misperception that our happiness and peace come from outside ourselves. Time and time again, I have heard patients say to me, in one form or another: "I really feel isolated and alone. I must be lacking something or I wouldn't feel this way. *If only* I had more money, or more beauty, or more accomplishments, or more power, or more status, or more fame, *then* I'd be happy, *then* people would love and respect me, *then* I wouldn't feel so lonely and isolated." Once someone sets up that view of the world, however, it turns out they're likely to feel even more stressed, alone, and unhappy.

Why? Until they get it — the money, beauty, accomplishments, and so on —

they're anxious: "I hope I get it!" The stakes go up, because it's not just winning or losing, it's being a winner or a loser that's on the line. They believe that everyone loves a winner and no one loves a loser, so they'll be even more lonely and isolated if they don't get what they think they must have. If someone else gets it and they don't, then they feel *really* bad, and it reinforces their belief of separateness, that we live in a dog-eat-dog world, a zero-sum game — the more you get, the less there is for me, you only go around once and so you'd better get it while you can. Perhaps most distressing of all is when they get what they thought would make them loved and happy and find out that the feelings of happiness and well-being don't last very long.

Paradoxically, the more inner peace we experience, the more we can enjoy life as it unfolds before us. In chapter 2, I described how important it was for me to learn to be alone and peaceful before I could be in a healthy, intimate relationship. Meditation was very helpful in my process of reconnecting with inner states of calm, of reminding myself where well-being really comes from.

When we can stay grounded in that inner, peaceful place, the paradox is that we can go out in the world and often accomplish even more, because the stress and anxiety that often get in the way are so greatly reduced. This is a very empowering realization. After all, someone only has power over you if he or she has something you think you need. The more inwardly defined you art, the less you need, and the more power you retain.

When we begin to realize how we set ourselves up to suffer, we can reframe our questions from, "How come I can't get more stuff?" to "What am I doing that may be causing me to get disturbed?" Not as a way of blaming yourself, but as a way of empowering yourself.

Fourth, *you may directly experience and become more aware of the transcendent interconnectedness that already exists.* You may have a direct experience of God or the universal Self, whatever name we give to the awe-inspiring.

Most spiritual and religious traditions are based on people who experienced God directly: Abraham, Moses, Jesus, Mohammed, Buddha, to name only a few. They did not *find* God somewhere outside themselves; they *realized* that we only appear to be separated from God. Their message was that the experience of God, of interconnectedness, of peace, is available to everyone via prayer, meditation, service, compassion, and so on.

Like peace, joy, and well-being, God is not something we attain from "out there" somewhere; we realize that God is *in* us *as* us.

I began this book with the theme that anything that promotes a sense of isolation often leads to illness and suffering, whereas whatever promotes a sense of love and intimacy is healing — that is, to make us whole. In this context, it is not surprising that healing is part of most religious and spiritual traditions.

When understood in this context, the realization of God, of our Self by any other name, is perhaps the ultimate healing experience because then we understand that we are *already* whole, we are *already* at peace, if we just quiet down our restless mind enough to know that: As Psalm 46 says, "Be still and know that I am God." We can enjoy, honor, and even celebrate our differences and diversity when we also experience the underlying unity.

Meditation is simple in concept but difficult to master. Fortunately, you don't have to master meditation to benefit from it. You just have to practice. No one ever really masters it completely, but even a few steps down that road can make a meaningful difference. It is the *process* of meditation that makes it so beneficial, not how well you perform.

Everyone has a hard time focusing, especially at first. Everybody! You are in good company. There is a reason why some people spend time in solitude trying to master meditation — because reaming to control and train your own thoughts is difficult.

When you first begin to meditate, you may find that your mind seems even more disturbed rather than peaceful. In part, this is because you become more aware of the disturbance that may already be there once you stop numbing or distracting yourself. Also, your mind may rebel when you try to discipline it. The analogy that is often given in spiritual traditions is that it is as if you have a monkey or a puppy or a child that is resting in your backyard. As soon as you try to train it, then all hell breaks loose. Similarly, the act of trying to control your mind can initially make it seem even more disturbed than it was before you began. That is a temporary process.

Some people find it easier to do meditations that are more active when they are feeling distracted. For example, you can do a walking meditation, in which you repeat a sound or phrase while walking slowly. Or you can do tai chi, or you can dance. Whatever it is that you do with awareness and focus becomes a meditation.

When I was severely depressed at age nineteen, I was in such an agitated state that I literally could not stop pacing around the room. How was I going to sit still and meditate when I couldn't stop moving? You start where you are and do what you can. If you can only meditate for thirty seconds, then meditate for thirty seconds. During those few seconds, your mind may wander a thousand times. Just keep bringing it back, gently and firmly, with the discipline and love that you would offer a puppy or a small child.

For many people, sports become a meditation. If you participate in gymnastics or diving or basketball or football and you don't pay attention, you are more likely to hurt yourself. One of the joys of playing sports is that it forces you to focus.

In my research studies, most of the participants reported much greater difficulty practicing meditation than exercising or maintaining their diet. Why? You have to eat; it's just a question of what you eat. Meditation, on the other hand, is not part of most people's daily routine or experience. Exercise is more familiar to people, and also there is a macho quality to exercise — you're out there really doing something, whereas meditation still has what some of our research participants called the "wimp factor."

From outward appearances, it looks as if you're not doing anything when you meditate. In fact, meditation is a powerful, active process.

There are many different types of meditation. It is found in all cultures and in all religions all over the world — because it works. Truth is truth. While the forms vary, certain principles almost always are found.

In most forms of meditation, you repeat a sound, or a phrase, or a verse from a prayer. Over and over and over again. You can focus on a sacred object such as rosary beads or a picture or icon. You can focus on a favorite prayer. It can be secular; for example, you can simply observe your breathing. In and out. Over and over.

Certain sounds have been found to be very soothing, and they are very similar in different cultures. These sounds are often translated to mean "peace," like *shalom* or *om* or *amen* or *salaam* or *ameen*. If you are more comfortable with a secular meditation, you can repeat the word *one*. A mother or father humming to their baby has an intuitive understanding that a humming sound is very peaceful. It also helps you to focus. These sounds usually begin with an "o" or an "ah" and end with an "m" or an "n": for example, "ommmmmmmmmmm" or "amennnnnnnnnnnnnnnnnnn" or "sha-lommmmmmmmm" or "onnnnnnnn-nnnne" or whatever word you are comfortable with. Inhale; say the word during your outbreath, emphasizing and focusing on the humming sound; inhale, and continue. The sound can be repeated out loud or silently, although many people find that concentration is easier when they say it out loud.

Meditation is effortless, and it is hard work. When you focus on something, sooner or later (usually sooner) your mind will wander. When you become aware that your mind is wandering and that you are thinking of something else, then just gently but firmly bring it back, over and over and over again. Without judging yourself, criticizing yourself, or berating yourself. If you understand that a wandering mind is part of the process, then you won't beat yourself up for not being able to concentrate because you know it happens to everyone. With practice, you will probably find that your mind wanders a little less each time than before.

This attitude of paying attention can help transform everything we do into a form of meditation. Whatever we do with concentration and awareness becomes meditation.

There is another kind of meditation called "mindfulness meditation" during which you

258

do not repeat anything. Instead, you just observe whatever comes up in each moment, without judgment. You just watch your thoughts bubble up without getting caught up in the emotion or the content of the thoughts, and then you watch the next one. You see them as events in the field of awareness. You just focus on watching your thoughts go by, without judgment, rather than repeating a sound. Both meditation by repeating a sound and mindfulness meditation both help to bring our awareness into the present moment.

One of the most helpful aspects of mindfulness meditation for me has been the realization that I am most often disturbed by people who remind me of my own lack of awareness. Now, when I find myself irritated by someone, I ask myself (when I am aware enough to remember!), "What qualities is that person manifesting that remind me of part of myself that I don't like?" Rather than being upset with someone and disturbing my inner peace, the other person's lack of awareness can be a great teacher in helping me to become more aware.

One of the most eloquent proponents of mindfulness meditation is Dr. Jon Kabat-Zinn, a friend who established the Stress Reduction Clinic at the University of Massachusetts Medical Center. We were having a delightful breakfast together one morning during a conference at which we were both speaking when a woman approached our table:

"Mind if I join you?"

"Yes, I do," Jon said, firmly but without anger. "We're having a private conversation."

"Well, I'll join you anyway."

"No, please don't," he replied.

"Here, take this," she said, thrusting a newspaper at me. "You just *have* to read this newspaper, *The Awareness Chronicle*. . . ."

Jon and I both laughed, realizing in that moment that our irritation with her lack of awareness of boundaries — her newspaper notwithstanding — was a wonderful reminder of those times when we, too, have acted mindlessly rather than mindfully and did not embody what we write and lecture about.

Here is a wonderful story told by Jack Kornfield in his book *A Path with Heart*:[34]

There is a tribe in east Africa in which the art of true intimacy is fostered even before birth. In this tribe, the birth date of a child is not counted from the day of its physical birth nor even the day of conception, as in other village cultures. For this tribe the birth date comes the first time the child is a thought in its mother's mind. Aware of her intention to conceive a child with a particular father, the mother then goes off to sit alone under a tree. There she sits and listens until she can hear the song of the child that she hopes to conceive. Once she has heard it, she returns to her village and teaches it to the father so that they can sing it together as they make love, inviting the child to join them. After the child is conceived, she sings it to the baby in her womb. Then she teaches it to the old women and midwives of the village, so that through-out the labor and at the miraculous moment of birth itself, the child is greeted with its song. After the birth all the villagers learn the song of their new member and sing it to the child when it falls or hurts itself. It is sung in times of triumph, or in rituals and initia-tions. This song becomes a part of the marriage ceremony when the child is grown, and at the end of life, his or her loved ones will gather around the deathbed and sing this song for the last time.

Imagine how intimate you would feel growing up in a family, in a village in which you were so fully seen, heard, and loved. My beloved and I cried tears of joy together when I read this story to her as the song of love expressed in that story resonated with the song of love in our own hearts.

According to one Zen master, "To be enlightened is to be intimate with all things."[35] As your meditation deepens, you may develop the perspective of the witness. From that point of view, you realize that you have feelings but you are not your feelings; you have a body but you are not your body; you have thoughts but you are not your thoughts; you have a mind but you are not your mind. You realize that you have these things, but they are not what define you. They are not who you are.

Beyond your feelings and your body and your thoughts and your mind is the Self that witnesses all of this. While this Self is beyond the mind's capacity to experience it, you can feel this Self in your heart as love: "Love comes from God, and everyone who loves is begotten by God and knows God; those who don't love, don't know God; for God is love" (I John 4:7).

When we realize that, this awareness creates tremendous freedom in making different choices. We can choose to live with an open heart, a love that can include everyone and everything. We are intimate with all things *as* all things. In that timeless moment, wherever we go, we find only our own kith and kin in a thousand and one disguises.

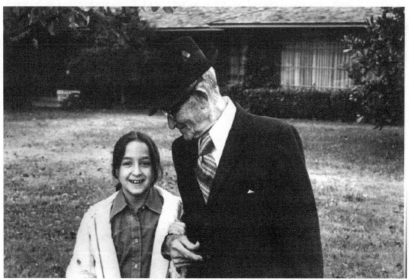
Grandfather and Kathy, 1970

5

"I Choose Life"

Jim Weinstein, M.D., is a physician with severe heart disease who, by conventional standards, should not have it. He has no family history of heart disease; he never smoked; his blood pressure and cholesterol were low; he does not have diabetes. He has very good genes: His father died at age eighty-nine, but not of heart disease, and his mother is eighty-eight, also without heart disease. Yet Jim was first diagnosed with coronary heart disease at age forty-six.

Despite cardiac medications, an exercise program, and the low-fat vegetarian diet I recommended, he was still suffering from worsening chest pain, especially when he got angry — which was often. While the changes in diet and lifestyle were helpful, they were not sufficient to relieve his pain. His doctor recommended bypass surgery or angioplasty.

He and his wife Rachel decided to attend one of our weeklong residential retreats at the Claremont Hotel in Oakland, California, near San Francisco. During a meditation session, he had a frightening visualization. He and his wife Rachel wanted to discuss it with me.

Jim: The image had come to me in deep meditation. The yoga teacher asked us to look at ourselves and imagine radiant light coming out of the top of our heads and our fingers. We did that the day before, actually, and everything was fine. Light was coming out of all parts of my body. It felt good.

But last night, the lights started

going out, first in my extremities: my fingers, and then in my toes, and then in my feet. Then the darkness started coming inward. The lights went out from the head, arms, and feet, coming centrally toward the heart. It was actually dark. I said "Whoa! What just happened?" The lights went out. The Hebrew word for "light" also means life. Darkness is death.

About ten days ago, I told my wife Rachel that I had confided in a friend of mine as well as to another physician that I had a premonition that I was not going to get through this year alive. The darkness and the premonition created tremendous anxiety.

On the one hand, I was hopeful. I read the copy of your book on reversing heart disease that Rachel gave me after my angiogram, and I said, "This is going to work. We're going to blow this sucker out of the water and reverse the entire process." But then, when the lights went out, I said, "Maybe not. Maybe I'm going to die."

Rachel: I had a dream in which he died. We were out west at a ranch. I was wearing one of those cowgirl dresses. In our religion, when a close relative dies and you go to a funeral, they tear your clothes to symbolize grief. In my dream, my dress kept tearing at this ranch. I woke up and I was crying. This was when he was having worsening symptoms.

Dean: I have learned that when patients think they're going to die, sometimes they're right. So, my first concern is the possibility that maybe you are about to die because of your premonition. But you experienced two different realities. One was one of light filling you up — radiance for your being, beaming. How would you describe that?

Jim: It was generally a very healthy, happy feeling. Something I hadn't felt in many years.

Dean: And the other image was just the opposite — darkness and death, which was terrifying. It was equally real. It seems that you are at a turning point where you can manifest one or you can manifest the other. And the choice is really yours. Why do you have heart disease at forty-six years old when your parents never had heart disease even in their late eighties, even though they ate a lot more fat and cholesterol than you do?

Jim: I always thought my genes would protect me.

Dean: Let's start by understanding when you get chest pain — what tends to bring it on?

Jim: Anger. There has been an ongoing feeling that I always have to fight to accomplish whatever I need. When I was growing up, I actually learned how to fight physically and emotionally. The fighting shielded me and it sustained me in my quest through college and medical school. My parents were Holocaust survivors, and their attitudes toward life were conveyed to me — how to survive in any situation.

Dean: Which are?

Jim: Rachel describes my constant presence as one of anger, but I never viewed myself as being always angry. I'm angry selectively.

Rachel: Jim, you get angry a lot. And usually, when you get angry it doesn't go away. It stays. You perseverate on the anger and then it . . .

Jim: It also solves problems.

Rachel: Does it? And if the problem doesn't get solved, you don't let the anger go away. You keep on bringing it back, you keep on fighting, even though in many instances we know that the problem is not going to be solved.

Dean: Jim, how do you see that anger solves problems?

Jim: Hostility has always been my friend. Anger has made me function very well and helped me to be able to endure a lot of the discomfort that medical training involved. In medical school, I was a pretty arrogant guy because the dean told me I was number three in my class in terms of all my grades and tests. I had a full Regents' Scholarship from New York State, and I didn't really study that much.

But anatomy was a nine-month horrendous experience. I loved it initially, but they gave us a surprise exam on day three — and seventy-five percent of the class failed the exam. Well, I had never failed an exam in my life. And that was sort of a jolt. After that, the only way that I could sustain myself through anatomy was sheer anger.

Dean: Anger at?

Jim: Anger at whomever was a professor. I said, "I'm going to show those son-of-a-guns." I was going to prove to everyone that I was not a dummy; and I was going to get the highest mark on the anatomy final — which I almost did.

Anger brought me greater focus and concentration. It also protected me. I was a very trusting, loving type of person when I grew up. The anger was something that I developed as a result of disappointments with friends and people along the years. It actually helped me to overcome the betrayal of some people who I thought were friends.

Rachel: Jim, you often feel the need to control things. Since no one can control everything, you get angry a lot.

Jim: I look for perfection. That's when I get angry, when things don't happen the way I expect them to happen.

Dean: Then it must be very frustrating for you since things are rarely perfect. Rachel, what do you see are the effects of the anger on Jim?

Rachel: Well, I think his pain and maybe this whole disease process is part of the effect of the anger. He only gets chest pain when he gets angry.

Dean: What about the effects on you?

Rachel: It does fall on me, and it's affected the whole family. Sometimes the kids are afraid to approach Jim about certain things because they're afraid of his reaction, so he's kind of unapproachable at times.

Dean: And that leaves you and your kids feeling alone and isolated from Jim?

Rachel: Yes. We find that a lot of the same issues keep on coming back in different forms. I've kind of grown to deal with it so either we don't bring up the issue or we have a fight.

Jim: Although people have told me that I have an angry-looking visage, I'm not always angry. Maybe I contract my jaw muscle so it looks like I'm angry.

Dean: Anger is something that gets conveyed through feelings. Even a blind person can feel when someone else is really angry. If you walk into a room and someone is angry, you know it. It's not just because of their face.

I want you to understand that to say you're angry is not a criticism or judgment of you any more than it is to say that you have heart disease. It's as much a part of the illness as your cholesterol or blood pressure. To the degree that anger or hostility affects your heart, then it may be worth exploring. The only judgment here is that Rachel and I care for you and we want you to get better, if that's what you want.

Jim: Thank you. I really appreciate your concern. Let's talk about an episode I had with a rabbi, because it's been causing me more anger than anything this past year. There was a point where the president of the congregation got up a few years ago at a membership meeting and asked why the congregation was losing membership and causing a financial strain on everybody. Everybody said well, other synagogues are opening up in the community, and people are getting older and they can't walk as far, and this and that. And everybody knew that was nonsense, because many of us felt that the real reason is that he was the wrong rabbi for our community. So, I got up at this meeting and I spent the next twenty minutes outlining all his deficiencies as a rabbi and his failures to our congregation and to the community so he would have no way to deny it. I totally undressed him verbally, and there was no way out for him. There was no way to deny it. I sealed all the ports for his escape.

The reaction was stunned silence. The rabbi's reaction was dazed disbelief. During the next month, we got together on four separate evenings over the course of the next month. His purpose was to find out what could be done to rectify things. And I said, "The best thing you could do is to just pack up and leave, the congregation is really fed up with your lack of abilities."

He said that he did not agree with that. And he said that's just not going to happen. He said the people felt that he was doing a very good job and that this was not a respectful way to handle a man of learning.

Dean: So, what happened in the years since then?

Jim: There has been a lot of tension and there have been occasional flare-ups. In the last nine months, I realized that he had become ensconced. He had become a fixture in the synagogue and I realized that I may not be able to get him out. So, I imagined having to debate with him and I visualized myself holding his heart in my hand, squeezing the life out of it, and watching him drop dead. It happened five or six times. It was not a daily image but it definitely concerned me because I had crossed a line. I no longer just wanted him out of the synagogue — I now wanted him *dead!*

Dean: So, you began to believe that having thoughts of wanting the rabbi dead might actually cause that to occur even though you knew rationally that this was not true.

Jim: It was a feeling that I could actually squeeze his heart and make it stop — which was completely unacceptable because my initial interest was to have my children learn from him. It was like the craziest thing I can imagine.

Dean: In your mind, however, it was real. And you kept visualizing it, and you haven't been able to stop doing it. What's the punishment for people who kill other people?

Jim: Well, death. Of course.

Dean: So, what's been happening to you?

Jim: I've got a death sentence going. What I wished on him has turned around 180 degrees and flipped back on me.

Dean: You've judged yourself already and just about executed yourself. While I might doubt your ability to wish someone else dead, there are studies showing that people who believed that they were going to die or who believed that they deserved to die sometimes did so. When did you first start visualizing his heart getting crushed?

Jim: In the last nine months.

Dean: And when were you diagnosed for having heart disease?

Jim: Four months ago. It's scary because I've never actually tried to physically harm anybody.

Dean: You may be doing it to yourself.

Jim: Yes, it seems so. The analogy is that if one of our children stole something from the store, what would we do? We would have them return it.

Dean: Would it be enough to just anonymously send it back to the store?

Jim: No. We would want them to make an open admission that they had done something wrong. To the person affected.

Dean: So, then, what is the diagnosis here, and what is the prescription?

Jim: I humiliated the rabbi in front of our congregation. And I left him no out. I have to admit that I ac-

	tually wanted him dead. I viewed him — and I still view him — as a block not only to my personal growth, to our family's personal well-being, but also to our community's well-being.
Dean:	Well, there may be a real opportunity for growth for you, your family, and your community right here with the rabbi. This man who you view as your adversary may be your greatest teacher.
Jim:	The prescription would be to try to make amends in a public forum.
Dean:	The sacred Jewish holiday of Yom Kippur is coming up soon — the Day of Atonement. Would that be an appropriate time to make amends with this rabbi?
Jim:	It would be so mortifying that I might even have a heart attack trying to do it. Maybe the right form would be in a room with the rabbi in private.
Dean:	If you humiliated him in a public forum, then you may need to make amends in a similar place.
Jim:	My friends would think I was crazy if I did that.
Dean:	On Yom Kippur, if you want to

277

atone for a sin against your fellow man, the Bible says that it's not enough just to ask God for forgiveness; as you know, you have to deal with the issue at hand. If I steal from someone, I can't say "God, please forgive me." I have to go back to that person and not only repay them but also ask for their forgiveness. You took it a step further, wishing the rabbi dead. What would be an appropriate way to handle the situation?

Jim: You have to get a group of at least ten people together and make amends to the other person in front of that group. It's not just for the other people's benefit; it's mainly for you.

Dean: These ideas are part of most spiritual traditions. Clearly, the people who came up with these ideas understood what healing is about. We're rediscovering their ancient wisdom.

You have a choice. You have two realities that are equally true, and you're right at the crossroads — your own imagery is very clear. You can choose life and light, or death and darkness. It seems that your disease became symptomatic after this all began.

My guess is that if you can stand up in front of a congregation and apologize, your heart may begin to heal instead of worsen. You might say, "I want to share with you something that I've done that I have regretted, which was to humiliate the rabbi in front of this congregation. I am here to ask for his forgiveness and for yours. Worse, when it became clear to me that I was unsuccessful in getting the rabbi removed, I even wished him dead. I feel terrible about this. I want to open my heart to the rabbi and to all of you by saying that I have done something for which I'm asking forgiveness — from God, from the rabbi, and from each of you in this congregation. This is what I need to do in order to begin healing my heart." Do you really think people would think you're crazy and shun you? Or do you think you would be modeling what is most healing and most noble? The words "heal" and "holy" come from the same root.

Jim: This plan would fit right in with everything I believe.

Dean: It's easy to write about these things, it's easy to quote scriptures, but it's not easy to live that way. Yet if one person can do that, especially a leader in the congregation, it transforms and begins to heal everyone. Not just you.

Jim: I might have a heart attack doing this.

Dean: Your imagery has made it clear to you that you are more likely to have a heart attack if you don't.

Jim: That may be true. The chest pains are getting worse — lately, I have been having chest pains almost every other day.

Rachel: We hear about it all the time.

Jim: Maybe I should go to another synagogue if that's the problem. You don't think that's an answer? Just run away?

Dean: You carry those feelings with you in you heart. Quite literally. You have to take your heart with you wherever you go. When you harden your heart, it affects you.

When we violate our own values repeatedly, our hearts suffer. It doesn't matter what *I* think, only what *you* believe.

"To err is human; to forgive, divine." All of the biblical figures messed up big time. King David fell in love with a married woman and sent her husband off to the front lines to get him killed. Moses lost his temper and was denied entrance into the promised land. Even Jesus had his moments of doubt. Everybody messes up sometime. We all fell down before we learned to walk. The problem is not that we should be perfect. The question is: What do we do when we are not perfect?

The whole point of Yom Kippur is that we all make mistakes. The entire congregation asks for forgiveness together so that no one can say "Oh, *they* mess up, *I* don't mess up." It's the essence of compassion: seeing what we have in common rather than what separates us.

Jim: There's no question that your analysis is right on the button. But

. . . there has to be another way that is as effective. I have young children. That would open them up to ridicule.

Dean: The young children may especially benefit if you can model how you want them to act.

Rachel: Jim, we're talking about you and your heart.

Dean: It doesn't matter what other people do in response to you. If it's clean on your end, you begin to heal. It doesn't matter what they say or do. Even if they ridicule you or crucify you, you begin to heal. To me, that was Jesus' most powerful teaching: If you show enough compassion in your heart, it frees you even if others remain in ignorance and darkness. In the long run, it helps to free them, too, but it begins to free your heart immediately.

Chances are, your congregation will embrace you and you'll have set an example that other people can then begin to emulate. You become a true leader in the congregation. But even if they don't, *you* begin to heal. It's clean on your end. You've given the power to make yourself sick to the person you hate the most. That's the irony. It's an empowering realization: If you are doing it, then you can stop doing it.

Jim: And this happens to others?

Dean: Yes. In my first book, *Stress, Diet & Your Heart*, I wrote about an incident that happened on the first day of my first study in 1977. Two of the patients hated each other. One was an elderly man who hated homosexuals, and the other man was gay. They started insulting each other, calling each other names. As the tension rose, I actually had to stand between them to keep them from hitting each other. One got severe chest pains, cursed, left the room and slammed the door, and the other got severe chest pains requiring both Demerol and nitroglycerin to relieve them. I thought that this was the end of my very short research career.

After they calmed down, I talked to each of them separately and said, "You're giving the power to give you chest pain and maybe even to cause you to die to a person you hate. Does that make sense? You have different choices that may help heal and empower you."

So every day I'd ask them to do different tasks to help each other like doing each other's laundry. Not so much to help the other person as to help free themselves from the anger and the pain. They never became best friends, but they both became free of chest pain. Their tests showed that their heart disease began to reverse after just one month.

Compassion can help free us from suffering. Not only compassion for the other person, but the hardest part is to have compassion for yourself. Those dark places in you exist in everyone. It's so much easier to project our darkness onto someone else, to split it off, to disown those parts of ourselves and pretend they only exist in other people. But when we can own and integrate that part of us — especially when you can do it publicly

— it can be healing. If you were to say, "Here's my darkness, and here's how far I was ready to take it; fortunately, I didn't die and I didn't kill anybody. I'm here to atone in front of you and to set a different example," then you begin to heal at that moment — whether they throw eggs at you or they embrace you.

Jim: This makes sense. I can say this is what my doctor said that I have to do to get better.

Dean: And if you want, I will be there with you, if decide to do it.

Jim: I'm afraid that I would drop dead right on the spot.

Dean: Well, I know CPR. You're not the only person who has ever wanted to hurt somebody, who wished somebody dead. Don't think you're so special!

Jim: The rabbi will still be there.

Dean: You can change congregations if you want. You don't have to stay there. You've done everything you could to get rid of him and he's still there. So your anger didn't accomplish your goal. You may find that you don't need anger to be productive; it often gets in the way. What makes anger seductive is believing that it makes you productive when it doesn't. It's usually *despite* the anger, not *because* of it.

Anger does help you to focus better; in that sense, it can help you be more productive. When you focus better, you gain more power, for better and for worse. But when you focus your mind using anger, it has negative consequences. Your blood pressure goes up, your arteries constrict, your platelets become more sticky and are more likely to form blood clots, all of which can lead to chest pain or heart attacks. Meditation and prayer can provide the power that comes from being able to focus energy without the harmful effects that anger often brings.

Jim: When I repress my anger, I get depressed. Anger gives me the sense of being Conan the Barbarian riding on a horse, swinging a mace.

Dean: I am not suggesting that you *repress* your anger; meditation and prayer, along with compassion and forgiveness, may help *heal* your anger. Chronic anger is toxic. Study after study has shown that chronic anger and hostility substantially increase the risk of getting chest pain, heart attacks, and premature deaths from all causes. So let's see if we can find another way to give you the focus and power and protection of anger without the toxic effects. A better alternative is to reframe it, to look at things in a different way, and to keep the focus and the intensity without having to use anger to drive it.

Jim: I pray a lot, but a lot of the time, because I've been doing it my whole life, it becomes very rote and my mind wanders a lot.

Dean: I'd like for you to consider using prayer as meditation. Focus on your prayers; when your mind wanders, keep bringing it back, over and over, gently but firmly, with real attention. Otherwise, you can be saying all the words but your mind is in Disneyland.

Jim: Exactly.

Dean: What you may find is that your fuse gets longer. Even when the situation doesn't change, *you* do. You don't have to choose between exploding in anger and making the people around you feel unsafe or turning it inward and making yourself feel bad. Things just don't bother you as much. Also, you retain your focus, and it's that focus that gives you the energy and the power and the intensity that feels alive to you. Otherwise, if you just walk away from things, you feel like a wimp, you turn that anger inward, and you get depressed. There's a third alternative, and that is to use the prayer as an opportunity to practice focusing. That increased focus gives you more power. You don't have to use anger to fuel that or to drive it. You can do it in a much more conscious and intentional way.

You will gain the energy that makes you feel alive without the toxicity that comes from using anger to fuel it. There are ways of motivating yourself by focusing in ways that are ultimately going to be more meaningful. Then, you may want to take it a step even further and use prayer not only to focus your mind but also to open your heart, which is of course what prayer is really about.

Jim: What you're saying is in the Bible: Open your heart. But I find it hard to open my heart to someone who thinks they're better than I am. Sometimes people of other religions think they're better. Sometimes people in my religion who think they're more Orthodox than I am think they're better.

Dean: Ego is found in all different forms. Sometimes religious ego is the most difficult. By ego, I mean that which sets ourselves apart from others. Anytime someone says, "I'm better than you because I'm more religious than you are, or my skin's a different color, or I have more money or power," or whatever it is — people have a million and one ways of trying to make themselves feel better or worse than somebody else — that is where suffering and illness often begin.

Anger closes our hearts; compassion is a doorway to an open heart. When somebody treats you badly, you can say, "What a jerk!" You can get angry that you allowed them to diminish you and then you begin to feel angry that you're buying into their view of you. The other alternative is to be compassionate and say to yourself, "How ignorant that person is." Keep an open heart, but that doesn't mean you necessarily want to spend time with that person. Surround yourself with people who have also decided they want to make an open heart their path, their priority, their value. You don't want to keep your heart wide open to somebody who's going to hurt you.

If you have no one with whom it feels safe enough to be open, then life gets pretty lonely and sad, and that only feeds the frustration and anger. When Rachel or your children feel afraid of you, it's hard for their hearts to remain open to you in those moments. Then you feel more lonely and angry, and it becomes a vicious cycle. Anger may have seemed like your friend but maybe the *focus* that the anger brought you was your friend along with the intensity of energy that came with that focus. Meditation and prayer may provide the focus and the intensity without closing your heart.

You may want to consciously choose to open your heart to Rachel. For example, you might say to each other, "I really want to practice opening my heart because I really want to feel close to you. I want to take our relationship to a whole new level. Who knows how long we're going to be on this earth, whether it's another year or another fifty years? Let's really see how close we can get to each other. Let's see, with our full intention, how fully we can be open and honest with each other. I want you to tell me whatever it is that keeps you from being able to open fully your heart to me. And I would like to really begin to examine what it is that keeps me from being able to open my heart fully to you." Start with each other.

Jim: I think that is very valuable. Rachel says that she is not as happy as she could be. I remember what someone once said: Divorce is like having a death experience while you're still alive. We're under a lot of stress now at home. At work, doctors have always been under a lot of stress. Now, there's also tremendous financial stresses.

Dean: I understand that — all the more reason to make sure you have a sanctuary at home so that you can come home and feel nurtured. You might say, "I may be right, but I'm hurting, and I can let go of being right."

Jim: I can let go of being right and I might be able to apologize to the rabbi in private, but in front of the whole congregation . . . it would mark me for life.

Dean: Yes. You would mark yourself for life in a positive way. You're not alone — everybody in that congregation who was there that day shares some responsibility by their silence. Somebody could have

292

spoken up and said something about how you went about humiliating the rabbi. Apologizing in front of this group allows them to participate in the healing. If that were easy then you would have done it a long time ago. Medical school wasn't easy, internship and residency weren't easy. Some things that are hard are worth doing.

For example, my program of comprehensive lifestyle changes is not easy. But it works for many people. I'd like to be able to say that cheeseburgers are good for you, but they're not. It's so much easier just to take a pill, but the benefits are more limited and short-term. Similarly, religion often asks a lot of us. At the time of the Golden Calf, many people asked Moses, "Why should I do all this stuff? Why do we need the Ten Commandments? Wouldn't three or four do? Why should we have any limitations? Are you sure they're not the Ten Suggestions?"

"Thou shalt not kill" was a radical concept for many people. It's hard, but there's a reason for it. It works. You could find an easier, watered-down way to do this. But I want you to take the high road, the hardest road, which is where the healing may be the most powerful for you and for everyone else by your example.

Rachel: Jim, it would be very courageous.

Dean: One reason many people are losing interest in organized religion may be because it often gets so caught in the form and the ritual while losing the spiritual essence that's most meaningful: the awareness of the underlying spirit that connects us.

Rachel: We talk about that a lot.

Dean: I remember a wonderful parable that I learned when I was in school thirty years ago. It's about a boy who was uneducated and didn't know how to pray, but he knew how to whistle. So he went to the synagogue and he started whistling passionately. People started to complain, asked him to be quiet, and began making fun of him because he didn't know the liturgy, he didn't know the prayers, he didn't know anything — he just knew how to whistle. But the rabbi was a wise man, and he realized that this was a heartfelt prayer. He was praying in the only way he knew how — whistling, but from his heart — which was much more meaningful to God than the person who knew all the verses but prayed without feeling, without focus, without concentration, without meaning.

That's what I want you to do — to go in front of the congregation and speak from your heart, and whatever comes out will be holy. If they reject you, then it's their loss. My guess is that won't happen. And you will be a teacher — a real teacher. The fact that you know all the scripture is wonderful, but it's dry without being able to put it into practice.

Jim: I can see certain members of the synagogue jump up and say, "I told you so! I told you so! I told you that he wanted to get rid of the rabbi!"

Dean: And then you just say, "Please sit down and listen. Yes, I had those feelings. And I am here to say that I am sorry. I feel very badly about that. I want our congregation to heal and I want my heart to heal." This could be a most powerful sermon.

Jim: This could result in a melee in our synagogue. Our synagogue is so torn and divided as a result of this whole rabbi issue.

Dean: It's already torn and divided. You're not creating it. You're talking about the prospect of healing it. And who is at the epicenter of all this? *You.* And who, other than you, has the capacity to bring the synagogue together?

Jim: But look what's going to happen. If I bring the synagogue together, then the rabbi's going to be there forever.

Dean: If you're not happy there, you can leave. Because your healing is all that matters. I'm not concerned about the synagogue or the rabbi, I care about *you.* If you do the right thing, when you start living in a way that's consistent with your values, your heart may begin to heal. Just like when you live in a way that's inconsistent with your values, your heart may get sick. Your heart knows. You can close your heart or you can open your heart. It may also happen that your healing also helps the rabbi and the congregation. Your own inner wisdom has spoken to you very clearly. What more clear and powerful images could you have had?

Jim: Clearly, this has become a life-and-death issue for me. And I'm not sure why it grew to that level. How did I get into this fix?

Dean: How you got into it doesn't matter. How you get out of it is what's important.

Jim: And am I in this fix in other areas?

Dean: I don't know. As you heal in this area, then other areas also may begin to improve. You may find that your relationship with Rachel becomes more intimate.

You grew up with two parents who had every reason to say that it's not safe to open your heart — they were Holocaust survivors. So it's easy to create a wall around your own heart that says, "If I open my heart, I'm going to get hurt. My anger is what protects me." That's what the wall tells you. It says that your anger, your hostility are what keep you alive and what keep you going when it seems like all those people are trying to hurt you.

The same wall that may have been necessary to your survival in the past is now what seems to be threatening your survival. We all need walls, emotional defenses. But the same wall that protects you also can isolate you if it is always up, if you have nowhere that feels safe enough to let it down — even your wife and your children don't even feel safe talking to you.

Jim: I never viewed myself in that way, but the reality is that you're right. Rachel has had difficulties with my anger and she says it's hard to get close to me because of it.

Dean: Do you want a wife who loves you and who is intimate with you or one who is afraid of you? Intimacy and fear are really mutually exclusive. Do you want to

	have a different kind of relationship with Rachel, a new level of intimacy? Do you want to move toward healing and intimacy or do you want to be stuck in loneliness and isolation?
Jim:	Well, suddenly the choice is obvious. I choose life.

Six weeks later, Jim apologized to the rabbi. He has had no episodes of chest pain since then, and that was over two years ago. His most recent tests showed that the progression of his heart disease was beginning to reverse. Jim and Rachel went into marriage counseling to help them learn to communicate better and to gain greater awareness of what causes each other to feel unsafe and to close down their hearts.

"Yes, my chest pain is completely gone, but that's not what's most meaningful. My relationships with Rachel and with my kids have become so much more intimate and joyful! I've been meditating by praying regularly from my heart — not as much as I'd like to, but more than I ever have — and Rachel tells me I seem much less angry. Yet I'm more productive now at work than I've ever been. I haven't needed the anger to motivate myself."

As a scientist, I understand that one case does not prove anything. As a human being, I was deeply touched by this experience.

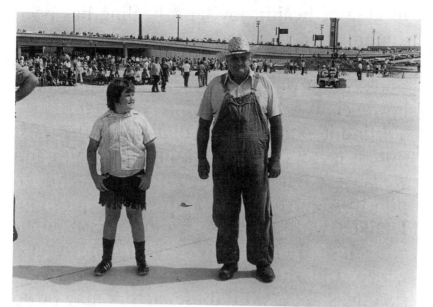

Opening of the Dallas–Fort Worth Airport, 1973

6

Dialogues on
Science and Mystery

By now, I hope that you find the evidence as compelling as I do that love and intimacy play a powerful role in our health, in our well-being, and even in our survival. The idea that loneliness and isolation predispose us to suffering, disease, and premature death and, conversely, that love and intimacy lead to greater health, joy, and healing has been documented by hundreds of scientific studies, many of which I have reviewed in this book. *Why* these factors are so important, however, is a bit of a mystery.

I find it extraordinary that one of the most potent factors in determining our health and well-being is so well documented and yet so poorly understood. To address this question, I talked with a diverse group of colleagues and close friends who very graciously and generously shared their thoughts and perspectives about why these factors may be so very important.

When I began, I hoped to find that each person's perspective might provide a missing piece of the jigsaw puzzle. And that is what happened. In reading the interviews, the picture begins to emerge more clearly. The pieces that are still missing are as interesting as the ones that were added, because they speak to the limitations of science and of intellectual understanding. We can sometimes experience and know what we cannot fully communicate or explain.

Everyone answers the question in part, but no one does so completely. In rereading the edited transcripts, I realized how much I learned from these conversations, yet mystery remains. No one can fully explain what is going on, why love and intimacy matter so much. Perhaps that is part of what is intriguing, for there is still so much to discover.

Many of these people talk about energy. While Western, allopathic medicine does not have a lot to say about how the flow and exchange of energy can affect our health — for better and for worse — this idea is a fundamental concept in most of the various forms of non-allopathic forms of medicine. Western medicine has not incorporated concepts that are now a conventional part of physics, such as Einstein's famous equation, $E = mc^2$ (energy equals mass times the speed of light squared). Paradoxically, this equation that ultimately led to production of the atomic bomb also underlies one of the most fundamental concepts of healing: In Einstein's words, "Mass [that is, matter] is merely another form of energy." According to many people, illness first begins in disturbances of energy that only later manifest in physical ways. In contrast, one of the most profound factors that enhances the free flow of energy is love.

I do not agree completely with what everyone says, but I find the various perspectives to be exhilarating. Some people are more reluctant than others to speculate beyond what the data tell us. Several of the scientists and physicians note in various ways that the current tools, models, and methods of inquiry of modern science are too limited to be able to answer fully the question of why love and intimacy have such powerful effects on health and healing. The question is not fully answerable from within the context of the inquiry.

By analogy, in most spiritual traditions, sooner or later one comes to the question, "If we are all interconnected, how did we come to think we are separate?" The usual reply from most spiritual teachers is this: That question is not answerable from within the context of the question. If you are in the middle of a dream in which you are being chased by a tiger and you ask, "How did I come to be chased by a tiger?" the question is not answerable from within the context of the dream. As long as you are dreaming, the dream seems very real, the tiger seems very dangerous and frightening. Only when you wake up do you realize the truth.

S. Leonard Syme, Ph.D., is a professor at the School of Public Health, University of California at Berkeley. He has conducted among the first and most important studies linking social support and health and has trained many of those who have gone on to conduct equally important work in this field. He is the author of numerous research papers and the coeditor of a classic book, *Social Support and Health.*

I asked Dr. Syme, "Why do you think love and intimacy are such powerful factors in affecting disease and premature death from virtually all causes?"

"I've been struggling with this issue now for forty years. My work has been driven not by ideology or belief, but by the data. In a sense, I've been driven to these ideas, because I can't explain the data in any other way — which is quite different from someone who might have a more spiritual or religious orientation. As an epidemiologist, I've been struggling with the determinants of disease, and I've come to this view because I had to."

Dr. Syme's first clues about the importance of social factors came during extended visits to Japan. He wondered why Japanese who had migrated to California had a fivefold increase in heart disease compared to those who continued living in Japan. "When I asked Japanese people, they all pointed to the social support issue. 'Westerners are lonely,' they said. 'Look at how they walk around in the streets by themselves.' " This led to a series of studies by him and by his protégés demonstrating the powerful role of social support on our survival.

"I returned to Berkeley and I found another doctoral student, Lisa Berkman, who is now a professor at Harvard. I told her my story and she said, 'We ought to look into the social support thing.' So she did the first empirical study of social support with a sampling from Alameda County, near San Francisco. Her survey asked some very basic questions, which I had used in an existing questionnaire done many years earlier, before I had any thoughts about these things. Are you married? Do you belong to organizations? Do you go to a church? The findings showed that people with the fewest social connections had higher rates of all-cause mortality over the next nine years, even after adjusting for all the risk factors we knew about. Her study started a virtual industry of thousands of social support studies all over the world. But I'm not going to get into any of that, because I have also now abandoned the earlier concept of social support.

"I then went to London on sabbatical to work with Michael Marmot, a former doctoral student of mine, who was studying British civil servants. He showed that both social support and social class were strongly linked with virtually every cause of death. We all have an idea of why people in the lowest social classes have the highest rates of disease: they are poor, they lack education and have bad medical care and bad housing, et cetera. Yet in the British Civil Service study, it turned out that people at step two — one down from the highest social class — had rates of disease twice as high as those at the very top. These people at step two were doctors and lawyers and other professionals, executives. They weren't poor. They didn't have poor education or bad medical care or bad housing, and yet their rates for disease were twice as high. So, we saw that there is a progressive, step-wise gradient all the way down the social-class hierarchy, and we knew this phenomenon was not easily explained. In all of the industrialized world, there is this same social-class gradient.

"So, it's not just simply poor education, low income, and bad medical care. There is something else going on — a greater control of destiny, which I define as the ability or opportunity you have to influence the events that impinge on your life. To the degree that you have more of that, your health is going to be better than if you don't. Since then, I learned that this concept has been used by literally dozens of scholars over the years, referred to as 'sense of control' or 'self efficacy' or 'locus of control' or 'learned helplessness' or 'sense of coherence' or 'mastery,' and on down the list. Everybody means slightly different things, but I think we are dealing with one common denominator. So now I understand what social support is about. *Social support works by helping people navigate through life.*

"How does this stuff get into the body? Most of the psychosocial risk factors are strongly related to a whole bunch of diseases that cross many body systems. Now, that offends normal biologic thinking. It's not the way things are supposed to work. Psychosocial factors like social support somehow tend to make people more or less vulnerable to disease, affect our susceptibility. Then, other risk factors — viruses and cholesterol and airborne particles and genes and whatever — determine which disease you get. If you are exposed to these other risk factors and you are not vulnerable, then you won't get sick."

As a scientist, Dr. Syme struggles with what he knows from his own experience and the lack of ability to measure these social forces. I asked him if he shared my belief that promoting a sense of connection, community, and intimacy can be healing, as well as quieting down the mind enough to experience an inner sense of peace, well-being, and connectedness.

"I am an epidemiologist. I really am data-driven. What you are saying really appeals to me at one level, but the skepticism and cynicism I have about this speculation is so great, that I have to say — maybe."

"Are the data that we have been talking about inconsistent with these ideas?"

"Absolutely not. I agree with you completely. You are just going one step beyond where I'm a little uncomfortable. I've spent my entire life trying to test ideas that everybody knows are true, yet ninety-nine percent of them turn out not to be. So, I come out to be a hard-nosed empiricist. I get nervous when I get too far from my data, because this is my life's work."

"Is it consistent with your experience and your beliefs?"

"Yes. I think that looking at this connection between relationship and survival is the most significant thing that can be done in our field right now. We are in a major crisis. We have tons of data with no theory, no way to connect all the little bits and pieces that have accumulated. We've studiously avoided speculations and theoretical developments to our detriment, leaving us with no overriding conceptual model. When we look at the data, we can no longer avoid that what you are talking about is the only way to make sense of it."

Jon Kabat-Zinn, Ph.D., is the founder and director of the Stress Reduction Clinic at the University of Massachusetts Medical Center, one of the country's first and leading mind/body programs. He is the author of several books, including *Full Catastrophe Living* and *Everyday Blessings.*

I asked him to explain the relationship between meditation, intimacy, and healing. "It has to do with a sense of actually finding one's place in the world and knowing it consciously, so you can navigate through the complexities of life with a feeling of groundedness and integrity — even in the face of constant change and potential threats to your well-being. I think there must be a physiology of that. I don't think we've even begun to tease out what the mediating factors are, but they are probably every bit as powerful as the fight-or-flight reaction."

I asked him, "How can meditation facilitate healing?"

"Many different meditative practices can help systematically cultivate a sense of intimacy, a sense of self-knowledge, vulnerability, and openness — a deep inner sense of tranquillity and belonging, of being comfortable in your own skin, of feeling your connectedness to the world. Perhaps such feeling states have their own biology. All of these things have, I think, long-term physiological effects, and possible health effects, as well.

"In my view, the experience of healing is directly related to the experience of being whole, of interconnectedness. When you taste that wholeness directly, it is invariably associated with feelings of tranquillity and peacefulness and entirely devoid of anxiety. There is no sense of a boundary between you and everything else, no sense of separation, or of distance, or of exclusion. No loneliness. It's like you are the entire universe, seamlessly connected with everything. When there is this sense of being completely at home, this sense of belonging or connectedness becomes part of your experience; it's not a philosophy, not a thought that we are talking about. It's the direct experience of this inner level of belonging, of intimacy, of peace. It's an experience devoid of worry about the future or the past. It's a total experience of well-being in the present moment, which merges into timelessness. The way it expresses itself in the body is phenomenal, because it's such a deep state of well-being, of relaxation. It's such a deep psychological state of connectedness that it is merciful, it is spontaneously accepting, open, and compassionate.

"I like to think that healing comes from a sense of being completely whole already. When you are tasting that wholeness, your body responds by restoring itself to whatever is the deepest homeostatic balance it is capable of. The physiology is in some way pulled along by this larger sense of merging with the entirety of the universe.

"Here is where a sense of compassion can spontaneously come up and allow you to see things without having them have to be a certain way. You can see the situation more the way it is, because you've gotten away from your own insistence that it has to be a certain way. And that can be profoundly healing, because your heart opens — it actually sees, feels, is intimate with and directly knows the heart of the other person. There's desire to do no harm, a desire to really nourish the well-being of that heart, that person, whether it is a child, parent, or lover.

"Experiences of the deepest intimacy can come out of meditative experience. From the outside, it may look like you are totally isolated while you are meditating, but in fact, meditation is a way to be completely in touch with the illusion of separation and isolation.

It brings an understanding that we are never isolated, never separate. In the yogic tradition, the image of a wave on the ocean is frequently used to convey the sense of the part being connected to the whole. The wave has its own separate identity for a short time, but at the same moment, it is a seamless expression of the water — of the ocean, of the whole. As a biologist I feel that way about life itself. Yes, life does come in individual packages: my body, my lifetime, my problems, my career, and so on. But all of that is, in some very profound way, an expression of life processes unfolding in an unbroken, seamless continuity of wholeness.

"Einstein talked about falling into the delusion of separateness. In a response to a letter written by a rabbi who was grieving the death of his young daughter, he wrote that separation is an optical illusion of consciousness, and that if we see things only in that framework, we become locked in a prison and lose the capacity to be intimate, compassionate, to know ourselves in the larger sense. I think that out of that delusion come huge amounts of grief, distance, tension — states that cost us greatly, by placing extra and unnecessary friction on the biology of our organisms. Ultimately, these states create the kind of wear and tear that encourage premature disequilibrium, disease, and death. I was amazed to find that Einstein would be interested in talking about liberation and inner security. His view was that the mind creates these ways of separating things, and so we miss the wholeness. One of his greatest trademarks was his complete commitment to seeing the universe as one seamless whole, and he felt that physics had to, in some way, reflect that."

I asked, "I am interested in learning more about what you call *inner belonging* and how meditation can give us the direct experience of that."

"If you are sitting or lying down, you begin to bring your mind to attend to the body. Ordinarily, we don't pay attention to the body, unless it hurts someplace, and then we pay a kind of reactive attention to the place that hurts, hoping it will go away. But the attention I'm talking about is more an open, accepting, nonjudging attention. We are paying attention simply to the breath moving in and out of the body, to sensations, to the proprioceptive [sensations from touch] qualities that come from the body — from the skin, from the joints, the toes, from the bottoms of the feet, the heels, all parts of the body with their associated sensations, which are constantly changing. From this dwelling within one's body, so to speak, very rapidly comes a deep sense of well-being. It's such a novel experience that very often people will have a flashback and say: 'Oh, I used to feel this all the time when I was a kid.' When you are practicing mindfulness meditation, you are tuning into proprioceptive experiences and experiencing the world in its most rudimentary form. You can learn an awful lot from that. That is what the cultivation of intimacy is — the willingness to be in direct contact with the actuality of your experience without judging it. Every time we judge it, we censor it in some way, we make it the way we want it to be. We get caught up in our desires, rather than seeing our experience more objectively. You can't have a direct encounter with your experience when you've already got a head full of ideas about it. The meditative work is actually taking off the lenses we usually see through, and just allowing things to be. That level of intimacy, I believe, is at the core of healing."

I asked, "Intimacy with what?"

"Ultimately with the sense of self, with who you are. It starts out with watching your breath or watching your body. Then the question arises — and it's a tricky one — Who is doing this watching? There is breath going on. There is the body and all of these sensations fluxing around. But who is the 'I' that is claiming to be watching all of this? Then, that 'I' itself becomes the object of awareness. The question becomes, where does *awareness* reside? What is its source? In the meditative traditions, that becomes itself the reflection, like looking in the mirror and asking, Who am I? What does it mean to be me to be in a body? And then not to confuse the name with the reality, but instead to inquire about what is underneath the name, that sense of 'me,' as in 'my body,' 'my headache,' 'my heart palpitations,' or 'my big toe hurting.' Then you gradually come to see what Einstein was talking about, that there is really no separation, and the very notion of an 'I' is a delusion of consciousness. We've defined ourselves much too narrowly. This is not some kind of psychopathology, though, abdicating the reality or usefulness of personal pronouns — I, me, my, mine. If you thought you were somebody else, you would be in big trouble. It's really more like an advanced familiarity with the whole question of what being human is really about, of who we really are."

"Some people describe this as having a double vision, seeing both the duality and the oneness at the same time," I said.

"That is certainly my experience. The tree

is just a tree. If you think that the tree is a car, you are going to have a big problem. You say, well, it's all one, so how is the tree not the same as the car? You can get into a deep philosophical argument about this, but, what I am saying is that the tree is a tree and the car is a car, and there is another way of seeing, in which both are manifestations of a deeper, seamless whole. We are all related in a multiplicity of different ways. Wisdom and healing have to do with understanding the complexity of the universe and knowing how not to be overwhelmed or eaten alive by it. You can fall into one way of seeing, be very stubborn, very blind, yet completely self-consistent on one side of the paradox — but you never see that there *is* a paradox. Don't you have the experience with your patients that they may start out very much in that conventional mind-set, and then, through doing the work that you do with them, their minds and hearts are expanded, and they have a larger sense of self?"

"Yes. That is often the most meaningful part of the work — for them and for me."

"I'm not saying that it has to happen through meditation. I'm simply saying that meditation is one reliable door through which we can choose to catalyze that kind of experience. I believe that when the body experiences that unity, where there is no boundary between the body, mind, soul, spirit, heart, and the world — when that manifests even for a moment, then something goes on in the body in the direction of nurturing or restoring it to its optimal functioning on virtually every level.

"Coming back to Einstein, we are more than we think we are. Our thoughts, which are highly conditioned by our childhood experiences, very often lock us into ways of behaving that may thwart the possibilities for intimacy. This happens in countless ways. We may be so preoccupied with ourself that we dominate, ignore, or eclipse anyone who gets close to us. Or we may be so terrified of intimacy that we only feel comfortable in a very restricted zone of emotions. Or we may develop a concept of intimacy that makes us feel good but doesn't allow for any reciprocity. When another person brings a unique history and feelings to the relationship, we may not be willing to tune into those differences, to become intimate and accepting of them. This might become a very one-way relationship, which ultimately will defeat the possibility of any true intimacy."

"How does meditation help a person change this?" I asked.

"By opening our eyes and our hearts. It

allows us to see the patterns of behavior that we fall into, and the ways those patterns create the prisons, or straitjackets, that have us continually falling into the same emotional reactivity every time we feel threatened in one way or another, or our vision of the universe is not being accorded the respect we think it should be. And then we lose touch with that larger sense of self and fall back into our more reactive, small sense of self. A lot of that is associated with fear — fear of intimacy, fear of being known, even fear of knowing ourselves.

"Meditation is like mining veins of gold from within your own being. The more you mine them, the more you follow them down into your own being, the more you discover that those veins of gold in you are also in every other person. Out of that, a greater compassion or intimacy for others naturally evolves. I've seen that happen time and time again for people. For example, there may have been certain ways in which you were disrespected as a child, because your parents had particular ideas about how you should be. You've grown up with that, and it's embedded in you, although you may have resisted it hugely and been very resentful of it. Then you have children yourself, and the same events come up that triggered the behavior of your parents thirty or forty years ago, only now you are in the role of parent. You might tend to come down on your child with the same insensitivity, hurtfulness and lack of respect with which your parents treated you and that you swore you'd never repeat. Those kinds of unconscious transmissions of thought and feeling patterns can create very, very difficult relationships between a parent and child. If you were bringing mindfulness to that experience as the parent, you would notice these patterns happening in yourself, even if the impulse is so strong that it's virtually impossible to control. Mindfulness is not about trying to control anything. It's about seeing clearly the actuality of events unfolding and not being judgmental — just seeing them. In this *just seeing,* especially if you are not trying to change things, lies the possibility of true transformation."

I responded, "In support groups for cancer or heart disease, people bring to light parts of themselves that have been kept in the darkness, because they thought those parts made them unlovable. It seems you are talking about using mindfulness as a way of doing that within one's own self."

"Yes. What you are describing is, what I would say, a group meditation. It's a collective experience of nonjudgmental, moment-to-moment attending, listening, sharing. That kind of group work is the external counterpart of what one does, by oneself, in meditation. Either way, it can nourish our long-denied yearning for acceptance, especially self-acceptance and self-compassion. Such a conscious group process can be hugely powerful, precisely because we *do* all live so much in the delusion of separateness. When we come together, and certain conditions are established so we are encouraged to feel safe and suspend our judgmental impulses, then we discover that this sense of connectedness has been there all along. We have a sense, all of a sudden, of falling into the experience of interconnectedness and are no longer feeling isolated and alone — it's hugely powerful. Then you are home. You belong. When you know that, even if that is not sustained (because the tribe, the group, the family doesn't get together in this way all the time), there is a deep way in which that knowing goes into your bones, into your sinews, into your heart. *Knowing* that you are not alone, that you belong, that there is a place for you, is profoundly powerful, and, I think, also healing. It's much better if it can be reinforced over time, but it doesn't have to be. You can have that experience of intimacy and connectedness even within your own body."

"What happens on an energetic level?"

"The emotions and the body are one manifestation of a larger whole. If you can come to accept how you are in any moment, it frees up huge amounts of energy that can go to healing. More than what is commonly called 'social support' has to be involved in healing. I tend not to use the term 'social support' to describe the kind of intimacy and interconnectedness we are talking about. It feels too outwardly oriented, reductionistic, in the sense that it asks: 'Do you have someone to help you get to the doctor when you have a problem? Are you a member of a church?' This is only one manifestation of social support. It's a useful monitoring of some sense of belonging, but it's only one dimension of a multidimensional world. What we want to ask about is the deep structure, not just about how it appears on the surface, even though the concept of social support is powerful and the data coming from these studies are important. To me, intimacy and interconnectedness have to do with meaning as well as with feelings, and with a deep sense of *who I am*. In other words, they relate to the whole question of self and self in relationship, all enfolded into intimacy and love."

I pointed out that in science, if you can't measure it, then it doesn't exist. Such questions as "How meaningful is your life?" cannot be measured objectively, only through the perspective of the person's own experience.

"Exactly. And this is where I feel science has to grow in order to answer these questions in a deeper way. A new kind of science — the counterpart, perhaps, of the Heisenberg Uncertainty Principle, and perhaps through the application of chaos and complexity theory, neural nets, and emergence phenomena — might help us understand how, in the domain of thoughts and feelings, we create a certain kind of reality. There needs to be a new vocabulary developed that would make sense of all this. We have to be willing to introduce a poetic imagination into science. There are many people who don't ask imaginative questions, but stay on the safe side where the funding will be. Then there are people who ask the deepest questions and just don't care about anything but what lies at the heart of their interest. Those are usually the people who are considered crazy by many of their colleagues, and very often wind up making the contributions that shift the paradigm and wake up the community to a larger way of seeing. It's not necessarily contradicting the other way of seeing — Einstein's physics doesn't contradict Newtonian physics — but, rather, expands it."

I told him that studies of Harvard students in the 1940s showed that how close they reported feeling to their mother or father predicted who would get major illnesses forty years later.

"These results are remarkable. They show how we formulate our basic views of ourselves and the universe early on. As adults, those views have to be looked at, or they can become like unconscious straitjackets we slip around us, keeping us from being ourselves. It becomes a self-fulfilling prophecy. That's why, very often in the meditative traditions, the metaphor is used of waking up. Because if you don't see how this happens, then you are basically living in a dream world that looks perfectly real to you. Everything you do will be consistent, and the whole world will respond to it, because that's how the dream goes. You can go through an entire lifetime without having the slightest idea that you were choreographing the whole thing, without any awareness that you had the power to tap other potentials of your being, ones you never even knew were there. And that's what I think we do in our work in mindfulness-based stress reduction, whether it is at the hospital or in prison or the inner city or in corporations — we clue people in, by direct experience, to the fact that they have vast reservoirs of untapped potential for transformation, and that they can slit open the straitjacket and emerge as if from a cocoon of unawareness, of dreaming. My sense is that you do the same thing in your program. There are thousands of different ways of doing that."

I asked for examples of ways to increase awareness.

"One way is by spending some time with yourself, without having any agenda, other than to be with yourself. If you can't do that meditating, another way would be to walk on the beach, listen to the waves, and watch what your mind is doing. Or lie down in a field and look at the sky, something kids do all the time. Go to the mountains. To give yourself a little time every day for non-doing is, in itself, deeply nourishing. Another way would be to listen to music in a way that is nonjudging, allowing pure sound to emerge. It doesn't even have to be music. To spend time in nature listening to sound is incredibly valuable, because it puts you in touch with how you are not really different from nature.

The hearer and the sound and the listening all become one — or they can.

"Take a look at the people you know — *really* look at them. Take off the lenses that you usually see people through. If I look at you and I say, 'Oh, yeah, there's Dean,' then I see you through the lens of how I think about you. But I could simply see you as the way you are in that moment, simply accept your being. This is something we suggest when we work with parents, to try to see who their children actually are, and to do that on a regular basis.

"The central core of mindfulness is non-judgmental, moment-to-moment awareness. It's not a philosophy or a particular position — it can be a way of seeing, a way of being, that you can bring to anything and that will help you be more in contact with the fullness of every experience. For me, it can come from running, from speed-skating, reading to a child, cleaning the house. There is virtually no activity you can't be present for, and, so, walk right through a door into intimacy and nonjudgmental, moment-to-moment acceptance of whatever is emerging in your being right now. That is fundamental. The forms don't really matter.

"Love is ineffable. Yet there is an approach to it that is very real, and we are groping for a vocabulary, a science to learn how to approach it. Intimacy is not just about love. It is also about peace. We talk about inner peace, but what is inner peace? It is that sense of being completely open — with nothing else needing to happen, including curing or healing. It's a total willingness to be at peace right now with things as they are. To me, that is synonymous with love, and synonymous with intimacy, and synonymous with the highest wisdom and courage."

Kristina Orth-Gomér, M.D., is a professor at the famed Karolinska Institute in Sweden. She has directed some of the most important studies linking the lack of social support to disease and premature death.

She describes her evolution as a well-respected scientist in this area. "I was very hesitant when we started out, because I thought this was a very soft concept which had a lot of problems in itself, especially in the research situation. But, I must say, I was surprised by the findings, because the findings seem to be consistent."

I asked her if it was fair to say that her belief has become stronger the longer she has been in this field.

"Yes, and especially from our recent findings, I'm surprised again. First, I was not sure at all what the concept was about. We started to ask, 'Is it possible to quantify, to measure this sort of very soft concept?' and second, 'What is really there?' The first question is — as I talk to other researchers, especially here at the Karolinska Institute — confronting molecular biologists who shake their heads and say, 'Oh, do you think that you can measure this?' That's one thing, and another thing is about the concept itself."

She described two aspects of social support. "The first has to do with very close relationships within your most intimate network, which is small — your nuclear family, good friends and maybe some relatives — whereas the second has to do with how socially integrated you are with your neighbors and coworkers; this aspect depends on your professional life, your social class or occupational level. . . . I think that the more extended network helps you maintain a better lifestyle, better health habits, and makes you more integrated in society. Whereas the other, the close emotional relationships, play a very central role for your own self-identity, for self-esteem, for basic trust. . . . One is what you get from your environment, and the other is what you give yourself."

I asked her to speculate about why social support plays such an important role in health and survival. "I don't have a total explanation. . . . I think it has some general kind of effect on susceptibility or resistance, if you like. If support is good, then, it seems, your resistance against lots of different kinds of disease will be good. . . . Social isolation seems to be the worst stressor of all. If you think how you react yourself to loneliness, it can be a very powerful stressor. What I think is happening is that it is changing the autonomic balance toward more sympathetic drive and less vagal [parasympathetic] tone." She said that some mechanisms are disease-specific: "There are effects of lack of social support on several possible mechanisms of coronary heart disease progression. For example, there is a strong relationship between lack of social support and low HDL cholesterol, which is not explained by diet, physical exercise, alcohol, age, menopausal stages or hormone replacement therapy, not even smoking. . . . We found that women who have lower social support have more and more severe changes of their coronary arteries."

In closing, I asked her if she was less skeptical and much more a believer in the power of these ideas than when she started.

"Yes, oh, yes, definitely. But, as you say, we still don't know the answer to the question 'How come?' Yet these things *do* make a difference, and we do see some of the pathways, that they do affect the central nervous system, the autonomic function, and so on. That seems to be quite clear."

I asked, "As far as you can tell, notwithstanding the important roles of biology and genetics, is this the most powerful across-the-board factor in medicine that we know in predicting premature death and disease?"

"Yes, even with the scientist hat on, I think so."

Gary Schwartz, Ph.D., is professor of psychology, neurology, and psychiatry at the University of Arizona Medical School and director of the Human Energy Systems Laboratory there along with his colleague and wife, Linda Russek, Ph.D. They are the authors of the forthcoming book *Love, Energy, and Health*. Dr. Schwartz shares Dr. Williams's desire to measure and quantify. The difference is that Dr. Schwartz believes that love *is* measurable and quantifiable, even if not objectively:

"I don't think these things are hard to measure. They are actually very easy to measure. All you have to do is ask people. I think it is a mistake to think we can't measure love. It's because we have the *a priori* belief that it's such a soft, fuzzy concept, we rarely think to ask about it. Simple questions about love can provide data that are very meaningful and important. In the Harvard Mastery of Stress study [described in chapter 2], Dr. Linda Russek and I found that simple ratings of perceptions of love and caring by parents obtained when the students were undergraduates at Harvard predicted their long-term health thirty-five years later. I don't think it's difficult to measure these concepts. I think it has been more difficult to define them and describe what they mean. That is partly because the concept is so wide and deep."

He first describes how a lack of love and intimacy can influence behaviors known to affect our health, risk factors such as diet, smoking, lack of exercise, and so on. "One plausible way to understand this is that the absence or the presence of love impinges on a whole bunch of mechanisms. They accumulate in a synergistic way. That would be one hypothesis. Now, that is the conservative hypothesis, meaning one that the scientific community could hear, and it allows us to say that the common denominator among all these risk factors is, ultimately, love."

However, other investigators have shown that the effects of love and intimacy on our health and survival are not fully explained by these traditional risk factors. He says that the impact of these behaviors may be missed because they are looked at one at a time, in isolation, when they may have a synergistic effect — that is, the whole impact is greater than the sum of the individual effects.

"It's not mediated solely through a single factor. And here is where systems theory turns out to be important. You start adding it all up, and all of a sudden, you start to realize something. Typically, the way our statistics work is that we try to isolate single factors. So if you have a small amount of depression, a small amount of hostility, a small amount of this and that, by themselves, these things don't do very much. But when you have the accumulation of all of these pieces, the whole can be greater than the sum of its parts."

I noted that even when looked at this way, changes in behaviors do not explain all of the observed effects on health and survival.

"Yes, there is still something more," he agreed. "The question is, what? This is where we get into energy — energy and information. The basic idea is a combination of two concepts. One is the concept of a system, which is when parts come together, and, through their interaction, they create a whole. Of course, that is the essence of the concept of relationship, which for human beings, is relationship with loved ones. When parts come together, and the system shares matter, information and energy in a way that is optimal for each of the components, and for creating a whole, then you have the most powerful and effective system. In other words, systems require sharing of energy and information and matter. You will see that this all sounds like love, once you start talking about it.

"The other is the concept of energy. In physics, energy is described as the capacity to do work and overcome resistance. It's power, or the capacity to influence.

"Now, if you look at the meaning of the word *love*, linguistically, it's interesting. I tell you, for example, that I love Linda. I love our dog. I love salmon with Dijon mustard and capers. I love the Catalina Mountains in Tucson. I love sports. Obviously, I'm using the word *love* in very different ways. I love Linda very differently than I love salmon. The question is, then, what right do we have to use the word *love* in all these different capacities — what do they all have in common? The thing you'll notice about how people use the word *love* is that they all refer to *a strong attraction or force,* a wish to incorporate something, to take it in. There is some sort of reception, a deep wishing to connect and to receive, when we love something.

"Psychologists use terms such as *bonding, attachment,* and *affinity,* and so do biologists and physicists. They refer to the essence of what enables a system to be a system, which is to remain connected by a mutually attractive force. When Newton created the concept of gravity, he saw it as a 'nonprejudicial force' that all objects of mass had, which pulled in all directions on all objects and interconnected the universe. He saw this *glue* that held the universe together as an expression of the universal love of God."

I asked him to describe the relationship between love and gravity.

"*Love is the fundamental attractive process.* It is the process through which you receive information. Therefore, love exists in all systems at all levels from the micro to the macro. For example, take water. You have hydrogen and oxygen, two separate molecules. They come together and they create this unbelievable, amazing liquid called water. What Linda and I are finally seeing is that what hydrogen and oxygen do, is bring out the best in each other. Through their relationship, they create something bigger than themselves, which is called water. The idea of love is not uniquely human. Love becomes, ultimately, very spiritual. There are levels of love from the micro to the macro."

"Are you saying that love is the unified field theory?"

"Exactly. What we are saying is that the generic meaning of the word *love* must relate to the notion of some sort of an attractive force. That is what we mean by love. Human love, of course, is far more complex than that. But it embodies the same fundamental principles. If *love* is the attractive force in the perception, then what we mean by *loving* is the giving back, the returning. It's the force to nurture, to protect, to care for. *Love* and *loving* are the back-and-forth relationship that takes place in all systems."

He then goes on to describe how love affects us via the direct transmission or reception of energy. "Let's make believe, for the moment, that love is not simply biochemical, not a molecule, not a location in the brain, but, in fact, it is a prerequisite for anything to exist as a whole system. Then, to the extent that a system can engage in a loving way, as an open, safe, and flowing process, in which all the optimal amounts of energy and information are flowing — that is what we mean by *health*. That's what gets us to the idea that love is the ultimate force — the *meta*-force. Our capacity to experience love is also the capacity to sense that energy at multiple levels, including the biophysical. That's why we are now doing research on not just the psychology and biochemistry of love, but the energy of love."

I asked him if, in summary, he is saying that someone who is feeling isolated, depressed, or lonely is metaphorically cutting himself or herself off from the source of energy or life or health — and that, in turn, can lead to illness.

"Exactly. The effects are first mediated through the known behavior and risk factors, and second, on an energetic level, through the direct transmission or reception of energy."

Joan Borysenko, Ph.D., understands human biology. She received her doctorate in anatomy and cellular biology from Harvard Medical School, where she cofounded the Mind/Body Institute at the Beth Israel Hospital — but she also understands the limitations of science to explain all observed phenomena.

"We can look at all the intermediary mechanisms between mind and body, but are they actually enough to explain the effects? Why does love often lead to healing, while fear and isolation breed illness? Candace Pert has a new book, *Molecules of Emotion*, that talks about the neuropeptides, which are important mediators of the mind-body connection. But the fact is, no matter how much we discover, at this point in our science, it will be insufficient to explain the totality of how our emotions and beliefs affect us physically."

She first talks about a conventional, Western idea: homeostasis, the need for physiological systems to stay in balance. "The organism tends to work very nicely until we put too many demands, too many stresses on it. I think where Candace Pert's work really figures in is that she's made it clear that the connection between the mind and body is mediated by the emotions. Healthy emotions have to do with open-heartedness. The true state of healing is undefended love. That is when the whole human organism comes into balance."

She quickly moves beyond a Western perspective: "We have to pay attention in our personal lives, and also as scientists, to the things that are mysterious, that we can't, in fact, explain. If we are going to look for the scientific mechanisms for why love leads to longevity, we're not going to find all of them, because we don't have any way, yet, of exploring the human energy system. If you go back to the Eastern systems and their understanding of body energy, the way the *prana* flows, the central part of what mediates the emotions is the heart. The heart center is the central *chakra,* with three others positioned above it and three below.

"What I think is going on from a mystical point of view is that we are all systems of energy interconnected with all other energies. Yet we have the capacity, through our emotions, to step down the amount of energy that moves through to us, which means we can cut off intuitive energy and we can cut off the life-force energy that comes into our body. My intuitive sense is that when our heart closes in fear — and our biggest human fear is of abandonment, that somebody won't love us — it decreases that flow of life-force energy. It just doesn't get to the cells and tissues in the same way, and we literally starve, because we've cut ourselves off from that larger life force. Every time there is worry, or fear, there is stress, and I've always defined stress as that which is isolating. Anything that takes you out of the sense of connection stresses you.

"If we open our heart, the energy simply

flows in and we are nourished by it. It flows in. And not only that, but it also flows out. An interesting piece of preliminary research about that is a pilot study that Dr. Janet Quinn did on therapeutic touch. She was measuring an index of immune function in people getting therapeutic touch, where the practitioner becomes a channel for life-force energy. This energy flows when the practitioner's heart is opened by feeling great respect, love, and care for the person they are helping. Dr. Quinn found that immune function increased in the person getting therapeutic touch, but it increased just as much in the person giving it. When the heart is open, that life-force energy doesn't end with us. An open-hearted person is always giving to someone else, and the act of giving is simultaneously the act of receiving. To me, that is the way that creation proceeds, when the heart is open to that life-force energy. We give it out in our creating, in our respecting, and in our nurturing. We also are allowing ourselves to be created and nurtured. Healing energy is something much bigger than the individual. An open-hearted person is always giving to someone else, and the act of giving is simultaneously the act of receiving."

I asked, "Would another way of expressing

this be that anything that creates the illusion of being separate, and only separate, fosters patterns of behavior, as well as direct effects, that may lead to illness and premature death?"

"Oh, absolutely. It all comes down to what I think of as the great mystical paradox. This is that everything appears to be isolated and separate. Yet most people have had an experience of being all one rather than alone. In a holy moment when past and future fade away, you feel a sense of oneness, gratitude and awe — perhaps what Einstein meant when he spoke of a solidarity with all living things. Or you have a near-death experience, and suddenly you perceive that everything is all one, everything is made of a matrix of loving, intelligent energy. Then the trouble is that you exit that state, and everything looks separate once again.

"So the mystic paradox is being able to hold that vision of oneness, that even though things appear separate, in fact they are not. Everything is united. To the extent to which people can make that shift out of isolation on any level, it leads to healing. On a physical level, for instance, hugging is a moving out of isolation, and if a person can really relax into a hug, it is healing. I think that's why the Chinese research has shown massage to have such good physiological effects. Any kind of physical touch, as long as the person welcomes it, is a way of moving out of isolation. So is volunteering. Through your very behavior, you are now connected to something larger than yourself. There is a wondrous emotional sense of being connected to something larger. It feels like a homecoming, a deep sense of rightness and belonging.

"There's an anthropological angle to consider, of life in the old tribal societies. Studies have found you can only recognize about three hundred faces — beyond that, you start to experience strangers. If the tribe got bigger than that, they broke into smaller bands. The way this relates to health and what you are talking about is when the society is made of no more than three hundred people, you cannot have many secrets. If you are hitting your child, everyone knows, and from within the community help comes forth so that you don't hit your child anymore. We simply don't have that because there are too many people in our society, and yet we have fragmented, at the same time, into these tiny groups, so there isn't any large group who cares for us, who can help us, who can be close to us like that. We have the worst of it — too big and too small, all at once.

"Healing occurs on many levels — but we will never heal politically until people, on an individual basis, are able to do the personal work of healing. Otherwise, we will get into a group, and we will project all our paranoia outward. It won't matter that we found community, because we'll find fault with the people in that community, and we'll put up masks, and we'll try to hide. I have always been convinced that we heal one at a time, and as each one of us heals, we affect the people around us in ever-widening circles, like a stone tossed in a pond. In this way, we bring more of a sense of interconnectedness and coherence to our life. We are not going to stop war through politics or aggression. We are going to stop it at the basic level of healing the individual."

Lisa F. Berkman, Ph.D., is chair and professor of the department of health and social behavior and professor of epidemiology at the Harvard School of Public Health. Along with Drs. Len Syme, James House, and Kristina Orth-Gomér, she has conducted some of the most important research demonstrating the importance of social support and community.

I first asked her if it is a person's *perception* of support or the objective *measures* of support that is more critical in affecting health. "It's both, and they are interrelated. Most people's perceptions are grounded in objective circumstances. We can try to change how people perceive things, but we also need to acknowledge that we live in a society where people don't pay much attention to the importance of being connected. We make decisions all the time — corporations, schools, city planners — and don't pay attention to these social factors which I think are very important.

"This is part of the reason why people in Japan and in France have low rates of heart disease. In France, it's not entirely because of the wine, although there may be something to that. Part of what may be protective against heart disease is that the French have a very socially cohesive society. I've spent a fair amount of time in Paris recently, looking at a cohort of twenty thousand gas and electricity workers in terms of social networks and work conditions. In Paris, at the unit I worked in, people go to lunch all together — secretaries with investigators. They all walk out together, sit at one or two tables, then come back together. I can count on one hand the number of times that I've had lunch with people in my home office, and *never* has everybody in our unit walked out together, and said, 'Let's have lunch.' Although the divorce rate in Paris is very high, the children still see their grandparents an enormous amount of time — statistics show that 50 percent of families visit their grandparents every weekend. So even when people are divorced in that culture, their families somehow stay more connected than ours do. I would name France and Japan as the two examples of countries which put a high value on relationships."

Dr. Berkman also talks about the importance not only of *getting* support but also of *giving* support. "I think the will to live can take people, especially older people, a long way. Actually, it's part of the reason why I don't talk about social support as much as I talk about networks and connectedness, because I think it's important that, in the long run, relationships are reciprocal. It's not always what you're getting, but what you are *giving* that counts. What often keeps older people going is what they can give, not just what they are getting, which is why the grandchildren become so important in France. When there is no more reason to give, they die. People make it through all kinds of stressful events. It's not just social support that does it."

Living in a strong community is not always

fun, even though it may be protective. Some people criticize Japanese society today and American culture in the 1950s as being socially cohesive yet repressive, with fewer individual freedoms, choices, and opportunities. Dr. Berkman's work indicates that a sense of duty, of obligation can be healthy. I asked her why this is so.

"Support isn't always a happy ending, a matter of what you can get, but more about being embedded in the whole social system — in a society, in a community, in relationships — that is important. This can be a real burden — but nobody said that the burden isn't what it's really all about. Because that is the sense of connectedness. It is an interrelationship that is both giving and taking, which is what love is about, what intimacy is about. It's not just about getting support; it's about knowing that you can count on somebody, and knowing that somebody can count on you. This runs really deep. It's not without responsibility and obligation and some constraints on people, but it's probably what makes societies tie together. It's this kind of network structure that is probably what promotes health.

"I've often thought that communities with very low rates of heart disease are also, in some ways, oppressive, conformist. You pay a price for living in these communities, one that goes against your independence and individuality. That makes it hard for people like you and me to be conformist. But that's what builds a community. It's like having kids. They take up all your time, but in retrospect, I would have made the same decision in a minute to have my kids. Or taking care of your parents when they get older. Because the intimacy, the love, the relationship — it's more than just getting things or having a good time. The meaning of relationships runs much deeper."

When I asked her why these social factors are such important determinants of health and survival, she replied: "I think it's very powerful in ways that we don't fully understand yet. I think this feeling of connectedness links to a whole set of physiologic mechanisms, such as the neuroendocrine system. It somehow involves stress reduction, and probably works on a hundred different levels. I think that there is no one answer, because it isn't a single mechanism, it's a lot of things. But, certainly, sympathetic nervous-system activity is one of them.

"Let me give you two examples that I talk about in terms of mechanisms, both related to heart disease. The early work we did showed that the *size and structure of social networks* were related to mortality, especially coronary heart disease, over the course of many years — as in the Alameda County study over nine years and our aging studies over six to eight years. We counted the numbers of friends, and so on, and we also looked at participation in voluntary organizations and religious organizations.

"The later work we've done focuses on who survives a heart attack, and the important variable there is *emotional support* — having someone you can count on. This is most strongly related to survival, and it's related to survival in the hospital and for six months or so after discharge. After about a year or two, it washes out compared to the earlier network measures. At first I thought this was totally quirky, but over time, I actually came to think there are two different physiologic possibilities going on. In the short term, for example, it can't be related to atherosclerosis or any long-term process, because those changes occur more slowly. It may be related to heart rate variability, to fibrillation, to some electrical phenomena. We are starting to look at that.

"Bruce Link wrote a paper, *Fundamental Causes*, in which he argues that certain things are truly fundamental causes, and they are not the proximal causes. We, as a society —

especially in medicine — are totally obsessed with the proximal causes, so that even in this field where the issue is so social and so inter-relational, what do we do? We spend an enormous amount of time looking at the biochemical, because that kind of research is accepted and is easier to get funded.

"I think connectedness and social relationships are fundamental causes. I don't think there is a lot that precedes them. I think that they are the determinants of poor health. There are other classic factors which are also fundamental and have to do with social class and poverty and discrimination, and a whole set of factors that travel together. And those two things are not unrelated. But, at the same time, I don't think that you can be reductionistic about social connectedness and social class. They are both important. I don't think there is something more fundamental than connectedness.

"When we think about how to strengthen networks and improve support, we need to work on many levels. Individuals should do what they do, like go to support groups if they need to, but it's not the answer for a society. I think that we, as a society, on all levels, need to think these things are important. And not that it's only important for health. I suspect it's just as important for business and corporations and industries. But *we don't even have it on the agenda.* For instance, there are lots of things corporations could do to promote connectedness that, I imagine, would even change sickness absence. In the same way, when we think about building houses, designing urban areas, public and elderly housing, we hardly ever pay any serious attention to the social environment. Housing could be built with more common spaces so people interact more. Part of what was so attractive about working-class neighborhoods was how accessible and mixed they were; old people, young people. I think there is a lot that medicine can do, too. You would hope that HMOs and managed-care organizations would see that it's to their benefit to pay attention to these issues. It ought to make sense to think about prevention, but for some reason they don't. Most of them don't pay much attention to increasing instrumental support (access to assistance and resources), informational support (access to information), or emotional support (access to love, caring, and concern).

"Let me tell you a story that kind of sums it up. I gave a fellow researcher and his wife chicken soup when their baby was born at home, and they sent me a thank-you note that said, 'I never did know whether chicken soup was emotional or instrumental support.' "

"Which was it?" I asked.

"It's the epitome of both. It's love incarnate."

Robert F. Lehman is the president of the Fetzer Institute in Kalamazoo, Michigan. The Fetzer Institute is one of the leading foundations in support of research, educational, and service activities in the domain of the mind, body, and spirit.

For Mr. Lehman, people who feel lonely and isolated are more likely to be unhealthy because they are cut off from spirit. "If God is the source of life, and if God is love, then love creates life. Every tradition has said that. What is healing but the renewal of life? All ancient traditions connect the spirit with healing, through love. Spirit is another word for life, for what animates. It has the same root in Greek, Latin, and Hebrew: All words meaning 'breath,' the breath of life. So, spirit is life. That can be taken in a psychological way, but why not a physical way, too? If there is a mind-body unity, then logic has it that when spirit is absent psychologically, then life is absent or depleted from the body as well.

"There are some recent surveys by Dan

Yankelovich looking at what people are describing as the new spiritual movement in our culture, and he's found some very interesting things. The number of people who say that spiritual growth is a significant part of their life has increased from 52 percent to 76 percent, while, at the same time, the number of people who say that belonging to a religious institution is significant has decreased from 78 percent to 50 percent. So, this is going on outside traditional religious institutions. But the other part of the survey showed that, of the 76 percent who said spiritual growth was significant, only 8 percent would identify themselves with the so-called New Age. So this is a mainstream movement that's growing rapidly.

"What is the character of that movement? It seems to have one or two defining characteristics, and one of the most interesting is that the unit of transformation is not the individual in isolation, as it always has been throughout history, but it's the individual in community, and the relationships which form the community. Relationships are the basic unit of the spirit now, and I find that very hopeful, because it's about becoming more conscious. Relationships help us become more conscious, and my own belief system says that when that happens, then love and intimacy and all those qualities become visible, and they, in themselves, carry an energy of healing, whether it's on personal, social, or environmental levels.

"My belief about this goes back to Martin Buber and others, in the early part of this century. They began to recognize that relationship itself was an entity, that there was an 'I,' and an object of the 'I,' and that there's also a space in between, which is an actual entity that has a spiritual character."

I replied, "In that context, all relationships are spiritual."

"That's right. All relationships are spiritual. That was Buber's great contribution, because he gave us the idea of relationship as an entity, that it exists. There's a German word for it, *zwischeukeit*. It caused some turmoil around Buber's reputation, because, at that time, people called him a mystic. But I don't know how mystical that is. Basically, it's common to most spiritual traditions. It seems to me that relationships that are open, honest, and conscious allow people to develop a level of intimacy with each other. They bridge the great divide between our inner life and our outer life. One could say by bridging the inner to the outer through relationship, there is a healing. This can be a healing between the inner and the outer in one's own body, the inner and outer in one's social situation, or the inner and outer even in the environment. I think, basically, it's where the spiritual dimension of what we are talking about comes in most clearly."

He describes how an intimate relationship can be healing: "What I've learned, both in my first marriage, in going through a divorce, and in a new marriage — and also in my close relationships at work — is that the way the spiritual dimension of relationship works is often by creating almost a crucible that twists and turns and tugs you, and pulls you into a higher level of consciousness. Maybe this is why relationship is absolutely the *sine qua non* of that, because you would never do that to yourself by yourself. [*Laughter.*] You have to be in an intimate relationship to have the kind of dynamic that's necessary to pull you into consciousness. And what happens when you become conscious is you begin to notice the projections you place on other people and things you're attached to, and the role of your ego, and you begin to recognize that what you thought was a darkness in some other person is really in yourself. You begin to see the wholeness of life, and in some strange, mystical way, when that happens the spirit of love seems to be able to flow in, and maybe your guard is down, maybe your ego has been brought to its knees. The spirit of love comes in, and out of that love comes a renewal of life. In my own experience, I know that if I wasn't in the crucible of relationship, feeling the pain and sticking with it, a good portion of me would still be asleep. At any rate, I have a better picture of my own wholeness now than I had in the past, and I think that relationships, intimate relationships, are necessary for that, just as crises in life are necessary for that. But in a way, most of us are in crisis all the time, we just don't realize it. A good, intimate relationship will help highlight that fact very quickly."

Rachel Naomi Remen, M.D., is the founder and director of the Institute for the Study of Health and Illness at Commonweal and medical director and cofounder of the Commonweal Cancer Program. She is Associate Clinical Professor of Medicine at the University of California, San Francisco, School of Medicine and author of the wonderful book *Kitchen Table Wisdom*.

Dr. Remen is a highly trained, brilliant clinician. While honoring the importance of the intellect, she also understands the limitations of the intellectual approach and of science to provide answers to questions that are the most meaningful. She was one of the first to write about the importance of meaning itself in affecting survival.

"It's the heart that adds the dimension of meaning to life. Without the dimension of meaning, life can become very difficult for us to endure. There are great pressures on us in the modern world, and unless what we're doing has personal meaning for us, we may not have the strength to go on. People face numerous crises in just the course of an ordinary day. Yet when we know that the meal we are making is for beloved people who will be strengthened by it, it is much easier to stand in a line at the grocery. Finding meaning gives us the strength to deal with frustrations. We can only find meaning by living open-heartedly. Meaning isn't a mental function, it's a function of the heart.

"The experience of the heart is what makes us feel safe in this world. When we can experience not only our own heart, but the hearts of other people, we feel safe. Feeling vigilant, feeling that we are not safe, we have to be watchful, we can't relax — there is a great stress in that. And stress is related to our vulnerability to disease. We are eased when we recognize the heart in those around us. And we can't recognize that other people have hearts until we have an experience of the heart ourselves.

"The more meaning we find, the less stress we feel, no matter what our difficulties are. I've seen this in my work with people with cancer. People undergoing very difficult therapies can go through them more easily if life has a deep meaning for them, and they know that their life means something to other people. A sense of meaning enables people to do things that otherwise no one would have the strength to do. So meaning is a form of strength.

"These 'soft' things turn out to be our strengths. It was only after I found the meaning of my work that I found the strength to deal with some of the pressures a doctor deals with and to go on. With joy. Many of us are living lives that have profound meaning, but we have not yet opened our hearts, so we can't see this meaning and be strengthened by it."

I made reference to the angel in the movie *It's a Wonderful Life*.

"Yes. And sometimes the angel is a disease. Sometimes the angel that brings us the gift of meaning is loss and suffering. You know, sometimes our heart needs to be broken open before we can know what really matters in life."

"Why?"

"Oh, I think we get distracted. Many of the spiritual paths talk about that. We keep running for the wrong goals. It's only after we get these goals that we realize they really weren't worth the effort to run after. Or, they may be worth the effort to run after, but they are not going to get us the deepest satisfaction, which is what we are really looking for.

"Many people who have had near-death experiences say that the purpose of life is to grow in wisdom and to learn how to love better. You can do this as a doctor or not do it as a doctor. You can do it as a street cleaner or not do it as a street cleaner. It is not what you are doing, but whether or not you are doing it with an open heart. That's what makes the difference."

I asked Dr. Remen to explain what an open heart means to her.

"The first thing that comes to mind is that it means the ability to experience that we are connected to other people. And it also means the ability to see uniqueness in every person. You cannot sit in judgment on something that is unique, there are no comparisons. I think that hate is not the opposite of love. Judgment is the opposite of love. It's judgment that closes the heart.

"At Commonweal we run retreats for people with cancer. Eight people at a time come and form a sort of a healing community for a week. I often wonder, What seems to matter here, what makes a difference, what strengthens these people? In any group session, everyone is having their own experience. Yet every one of these people knows that their life matters to the others. In some way that can't be measured, knowing our lives matter to others seems to strengthen the will to live in us. It enables us to value our lives, because we see that value reflected back from others. They may not always agree with everything that we are saying, but *who we are* is important to them. Our life matters, our suffering matters. It is so hard to find this kind of relationship in our society. The message we get is that we *don't* matter. But every human life matters. We all suffer in ways as unique as our fingerprints, but we are all *capable* of suffering. I think that vulnerability, that shared vulnerability, is what matters. There is no one, no matter how wealthy, how brilliant, how famous, who is not capable of suffering. Therefore, no one is alone in their suffering and every one is capable of understanding that suffering. Capable of compassion. Suffering is the great teacher of compassion."

"And being vulnerable is a doorway to intimacy."

"Yes. And intimacy heals suffering. We suffer not because we're in pain. The real suffering is that we feel we are in pain *alone*. That is what this particular culture does. It isolates us from each other so that people think they're alone. So many people have come to me and said, 'You know, this is happening to me'. . . and, as they tell the story of what has happened to them, it's as if they believe that they are the only one feeling such a thing. Other people are happy, other people would not understand how it was for them. We all wear masks that hide our true nature. We don't even recognize that we are not in this alone. We simply couldn't bear it, if we really were in it alone."

So, once again, we returned to the fundamental question, "Why does a sense of isolation so profoundly affect our survival and our health?"

"There is a factor in here that's difficult to measure. We might talk about it as the will to live, an unknown factor which enables people to mobilize their physiology, to deal with obstacles and push through physical difficulties. We look to science to explain why some people get well and some people don't get well. But I think there may be something else far more mysterious in our ability to recover than simply having the right treatment or the right surgery. There are people who get well when their physicians think they have no business getting well. There are people who don't get well who seem to have had every chance to recover. Perhaps something about knowing that others care, that your suffering matters to other people, your joy matters to other people, *you* matter to other people — that strengthens this deep impulse toward life that is in every one of us. We find this in community and in intimacy. Being loved is kind of a grace. It's not earned. It's just somebody reflecting back that this little life that we have, this single human being, makes a difference in this world. Something about that activates this dimension in us that is able to fight for that life, because it matters. So much in our culture tends to erase our uniqueness. We're just a number, we're invisible people."

I asked her to explain why studies have shown that as little as six weeks in a loving, supportive group can affect recurrence and death rates from cancer years later.

"Perhaps once you've been seen, once you know that your life matters to someone, it can't be taken back. It's an all-or-nothing phenomenon. You do not need to be with the people to whom your life matters. You just need to know that there is someplace in this world that you matter. Either you are seen or you are not seen; either you know you matter or you don't. Experiencing it, not just being told it. Once that happens, you have that strength forever. Perhaps that is why good parenting is so important. You discover that you are loved as you are. Many people have never been loved whole."

I asked, "Because they have nowhere that feels safe enough to let their walls down to open their hearts, and no one they feel close enough to do that with?"

"We fear judgment. Or abandonment. In many of the cancer groups, people are talking about things that have caused other people to judge them or abandon them. Many times people have discovered that some of their friends are gone in hard times, once they have cancer. But instead of distancing, the group gets closer. And it is not about sitting around and whining about your problems. Every cancer group is a group of warriors, people who have become strong enough through their own suffering to hear anything and not worry. Strong enough to love others without fear of loss. That gives every person there the opportunity to be who they are and be cared about exactly as they are. Most of us have never experienced that.

"Just listening to people generously strengthens them, because then they can become more fully present. They are not trying to keep parts of themselves out of the room. They can be there in one piece. As you listen to someone, they stop fixing themselves in order to get approval, and remember who they are. Anything that has been fixed is not as strong as something that is whole. We have learned to become ashamed of our wholeness in this culture. There are parts of ourselves that we are ashamed of, that we hide, which are the very parts we may need in order to recover — either to recover from an illness or to live well with an illness. Anything that is not intellectual is seen as a weakness in this culture — the intuition, the spirit, the soul, the heart. Up until very recently, people devalued these things. It still opens one up to the pointing finger of *touchy-feely*. But I don't care about that pointing finger anymore. Often the people who point that finger have no idea what human strength looks like, or what human power looks like. These things that are seen as so soft are far more powerful, when the chips are down, than the ideas and the intellect, all these things we respect so much. They are what enable us to meet with the events of our lives and not be trampled by them.

Ideas are not as powerful as the heart and the soul. Love is more powerful than ideas.

"It is our vulnerability that makes us lovable, that allows other people to feel safe enough to open their hearts to us. What we are really looking for is not approval, but intimacy, acceptance — which comes from vulnerability, not from perfection. It is the power of our vulnerability. It doesn't make sense, it's just real. Many things which are real do not make sense to the mind. But it's the way that the world works anyway. The mind is only one way of processing life. And that is the great secret here in Western culture, that many of the things that don't make sense are what are most real. Things that can't be measured are most real, most valuable. Things that can't be proven can become the foundation of a better life.

"So we end up with a paradox — the realization that by accepting our vulnerability, we can become more than we ever dreamed possible. That it isn't our perfection which allows us to fulfill our potential, but our vulnerability that allows us to become fulfilled. Even when we can't fix a problem, we can grow larger than the problem, so that the problem becomes a smaller and smaller part of the totality we are."

I asked her about the transformational

value of suffering — what is transforming into what?

"There is something about human consciousness that has the capacity to transform pain into wisdom. It's possible to live a very good life, even though it isn't an easy life. We can fulfill the purpose of life whether we are sick or well. To grow in wisdom and to learn to love better."

Sri Swami Satchidananda is the founder and director of the Integral Yoga Institutes and of the Light of Truth Universal Shrine (LOTUS) in Buckingham, Virginia, which is an ecumenical shrine dedicated to finding common ground among the world's religions. He is a renowned spiritual leader who has dedicated his life to the cause of peace — both individual and universal. I have been fortunate to study with him for more than twenty-five years.

Not surprisingly, Swami Satchidananda brings an overtly spiritual perspective to explain why love and intimacy affect our health and survival. When I asked him why loneliness and isolation predispose people to illness, he replied on different levels. On the psychological level, he said, "When there is no one they can communicate with and share their problems with, they bottle it up in themselves. When they talk to someone else, they are sharing their burden, so the burden is reduced, halved. Your body is a mirror of your mind, a product of your own mind. Although you only see the face, every cell expresses it. The whole body changes according to your thoughts and emotions. A happy mind will make a happy body, a healthy body. When people feel lonely and unhappy, their whole body changes. It loses its immunity. Anything that disturbs the mind causes problems."

He distinguished between being alone and being lonely. "Lonely means you are forced to be alone. You can *choose* to be alone, and it's quite different. Everybody can have company with one's Self, with the God within. You can talk with the 'still small voice within.' But not everyone can do that at first. They need to have company with people, somebody to share with. When they share, their burden is lessened. They feel comfortable, so they are healthy. But it is not the ultimate solution. Relationships also can create dependency. It is temporary. There is also company with what you call higher consciousness — the God in you. You can communicate with that. The individual mind talks to a higher mind. . . . Nobody is actually truly isolated. You have company within you. You don't realize it. This is what we call ignorance of one's own Self. . . . I enjoy being by myself, *and* I enjoy being around other people. I don't *depend* on other people being around for my happiness."

When I asked, "What is the root of healing?" he replied, "Contentment. Contentment comes by quieting down the mind and body enough — whether through meditation, yoga, or prayer — to experience an inner sense of peace and joy and well-being, and, ultimately, to experience God within. It doesn't mean that you should not love anybody. Love for love's sake, but don't depend on that. In one of the Upanishads, the husband loves the wife not for the sake of the wife, but for the sake of love. You love the Self in her."

"So, if I can love the Self in her, then I can love the Self in me, and then, ultimately, I can see them as one and the same?"

"That's right. Then you won't feel separate. You realize that you are loving yourself through your beloved, and then you will learn to love everybody the same way, because you are truly loving yourself. You can never be separated from your own true Self. There may be dozens of people around you, or you are all alone, but it's always the same you."

★ ★ ★

Robert A. F. Thurman is the Jey Tsong Khapa Professor of Indo-Tibetan Studies at Columbia University and one of the most well-known exponents of Tibetan Buddhism. He was chosen by *Time* magazine as one of the fifty most influential Americans in 1997.

He began our discussion by saying, "The human life form — and that of mammals, in general — is very much based on the possibility of overcoming the boundary of self and other. By taking the young inside your own body, you actually break the perimeter of the skin and have a visceral experience there. . . . Only at a certain point later in life do you actually differentiate it as a separate being. . . .

"The human life form itself is a very interconnected life form. Its life depends upon being aware of other beings. Its natural state is to be interactive with siblings and family, because it comes out of its mother's womb, where it spends a long time, and then it stays in close contact with its parents again for a long time, in order to grow up safely. So, due to all of these factors, if a human being comes into an unnatural state of being very much by itself over a long period of time, it's like a death. It is natural that the being would lose meaning or purpose in life, and become depressed and discouraged, and that their bodily systems wouldn't work well, because they would have such a low sense of self."

As a Buddhist, Professor Thurman is a proponent of reincarnation. According to him, even the desire to seek another birth derives from the suffering that comes from the experience of being alone after death. "The time of ultimate loneliness, in the Buddhist perspective, is at the moment of death. . . . In fact, death is defined as the moment of severance from all relationships. Precisely because it is so used to being embedded in relationships, that being seeks rebirth, a new embodiment, so it can have a new nexus of interconnectedness."

Like Swami Satchidananda, Professor Thurman distinguishes loneliness from being alone. "I would say that *loneliness* — meaning the feeling that no one cares for you and you don't care for anyone else, of being shut off from people rather than simply being alone — that is the worst thing. Some saints, like St. Francis or Milarepa, could be quite alone in a Himalayan cave with just a few birds, but they would feel connected to all human beings. They would even value the aloneness as a means to broaden their sense of relatedness to everybody. So, I think it has to do with the attitude."

He goes on to say that it's not just a question of aloneness. "From a Buddhist perspective, I think one would say that it is a question of the presence or absence of lovingness. Loving, of course, is a way of positively connecting with others. Buddhism defines love as willing or wanting the happiness of another. That is real love, as distinct from desire, which could be possessive, as in wanting to experience pleasure from possessing another. But true love just wants the other to be happy, there's that wish for the other to be happy, and the Buddhists have this funny paradox, where in forgetting about yourself, being absorbed in desiring the happiness of another — that's when you have the highest happiness. . . .

"Whether you happen to be with people or apart from people, if you feel loving toward them, then you will feel happiness. If you feel angry toward them and disgusted with them, then you will feel unhappy. Maybe, instead of loneliness, it should be labeled a state of isolation, a state of disaffection, as opposed to a state of vibrant lovingness. I think lovingness is actually the key."

In other words, compassion can be healing. "The experience of broadening one's sense of identity to incorporate another is maybe the key to what is healing. It creates a broader pool of energy where you feel more energized by relating with another, rather than being locked up in yourself. . . . Suffering is based on ignorance or lack of awareness. . . . Ignorance is not only the ignorance of not knowing some fact, like how many fish are in the ocean. It's ignorance about your own existential situation, the delusion that you are a separate being from the world, the most important thing in the world and the only real thing in the world, and that other things are dubious. . . . We are always in some struggle with the world, which we perceive as different from ourselves. That is the fundamental ignorance. It's the lack of awareness of the relative, temporary, and fluctuating difference between self and other, seeing instead some absolute difference between self and other. It fits perfectly with your theme, which is that the more aware you are of your interconnectedness with the universe, the stronger and healthier you are, while the more solidified you are about the idea you are some unique, special, separate thing, the more sick you are. The whole source of illness from the Buddhist perspective is just that."

I asked, "Then the essence of healing is to maintain a double vision, which sees on one level that we are separate, while on another level, we are a part of everything?"

He replied, "Absolutely. That is quite true, although to break out of the cage of feeling separate and alienated from the world, the emphasis, at a certain stage, is on finding oneness with the world, seeing beyond the illusion of separateness. Once, however, one discovers interconnectedness with the rest of the world, one has a second stage of redefining a healthy separateness — not exaggerated but a healthy individuality — which is based on the double vision, as you say. But you can't jump to the double vision instantly; you have to first critique strongly the sense of self-separation and isolation, and then have the melting experience of yourself as one with the universe. Once you have had that, though, you don't want to get stuck in it. You would just become a piece of glop. This can happen to some people. Instead, you have to then redefine yourself, but now as a conscious, creative act. That is when you add the other component of the double vision."

I asked him what we can do to overcome feelings of being separate and only separate.

"There is active meditation, working

meditation — not just walking around in a zendo, but walking out into the streets. Go and do some work in the homeless shelter. Go out and do what Roshi Glassman calls 'street retreats.' Go out and help somebody, cook some lunch for some homeless person. Go to some hospital and play with the bambinos. Read a book to a kid who has cancer. Do some sort of a meditation where you get out, force yourself to interact and find out how health-giving it is to care for somebody. I think doing that kind of social thing is really important. Look at Princess Diana and Mother Teresa, and the great lesson it's been for the planet, how in their lives and in their passing, they showed us that people really do appreciate loving and caring. Look at the outpouring of people's feelings after they died."

Carol Naber is an intuitive healer who lives in northern California. I asked her perspective on the role of love and survival.

"It's the *perception* of loneliness that matters, because the reality of our existence is we are all connected, we are never really alone. The perception of loneliness is not the truth, but our egos often dictate the realities that we perceive. The heart is all about relationship. You don't feel lonely if you're in a relationship to yourself, to your environment, to God, to people. The key to healing is having an open heart.

"Healing energy is always available. It surrounds us. But our hearts must be open to receive what is available. I can't heal if my heart isn't open. I can't access that healing energy. If you are feeling angry, you are blocking that flow, you are shut down. You are, in fact, cutting yourself off from connection, and the energy gets stuck, it stops flowing. Disease often first begins in the energetic field — the aura — and only later may manifest physically. When your energy flows, it regenerates your aura and then goes to help heal the body.

"Anger is often a manifestation of other emotions, like fear and shame. Perhaps more than any other emotion, shame keeps us from connecting. Shame is about hiding that part of ourselves we are so afraid to bring up, because we believe that if anyone found out about it, they'd never love us or want to be around us. It's so much more acceptable to bring up anger, or sadness, or even fear. We've learned how to hide our shame, to keep it at bay, so we don't bring it up in our relationships. But one of the most healing things you can do — and this is why I'm so interested in safe, group environments for healing — is to bring up those parts, to disclose them. How much more connected and intimate you feel with others when you can bring up the most shameful parts of yourself and find that they don't run away!

"The key for healing is relationship. Being loved is about being seen, having a safe enough place to express yourself, to express your feelings. When somebody is willing to hear you, to even repeat back what they've heard you say, it can feel like an amazing, loving act. When you really feel like you are being heard, then you feel seen. To feel seen is to feel connected. In that context, listening is a spiritual practice. I don't know that is even necessary to always see the commonality. You just have to be able to see into a person deeply enough so you can recognize something and mirror it back. For example, a person might be very upset, and you don't have to see the same aspect in yourself. You can just say, 'It sounds like you are really upset,' and they will feel seen and heard. In my work, the healing that happens is in the heart connection, in bearing witness to someone's journey so they are not all by themselves. My whole task is to make sure that people are feeling seen."

I asked, "Why is feeling seen and feeling connected healing?"

"Because it opens your heart, the core energy place. I don't know if I fully understand it, but it expands both of us, and it resonates us to something larger, one which is more in line with how our bodies need to vibrate and resonate. It's an energy in the universe that is beyond us, while it's also within us.

"We're separate and we're not separate. We all embody the whole universe, each one of us, yet we're also separate. But, like a hologram, you can find the whole within each of the separate pieces. Healing is a journey, and we can experience it through our relationships with others."

John Gray, Ph.D., is the author of several books, including *Men Are from Mars, Women Are from Venus*. He has had extensive experience helping people increase the level of intimacy in their relationships. I asked him to provide his perspective on why intimacy is so important.

"When people do not experience intimacy, do not experience a relationship, do not experience love on a spiritual level, then they are disconnected from who they are as spiritual beings, from what they are here to do in this world. I feel there is a spiritual purpose, a direction that we have as human beings, which is to love and be loved. Who we are, in truth, is a simple fact of who every person is, a loving being. When we are not expressing ourselves in situations which allow us to be loving, which allow us to feel loved, to nurture and be nurtured in that way, then we are disconnected from who we are. And when this happens, we are disconnected from the source of happiness, the source of aliveness. We feel emotions and attitudes that are not really our true selves. Therefore, we seek escape from this non-self state, this suffering. When you are aligned with who you truly are, you don't experience suffering. You may experience pain. If you lose someone, you are going to experience pain, but you are not going to suffer to the same degree and in the same way. It's a different kind of experience, and you move through it."

Like Dr. Rachel Remen, he described the importance of meaning in enhancing our will to live. "Having children gives a sense of meaning and direction and purpose in life. It makes you love your life. If your life doesn't have meaning, you don't love it. You kind of wonder, 'Why am I even here? Why do I put up with these problems?' Your health is certainly going to be a reflection of your answer to the question, Do I want to be alive? Do I love my life? People who live long and happily love their lives. People who don't, in many cases, die, because some part of them doesn't love their life. They don't want to be alive. You can see the death urge being very strong in a lot of people who have premature death, or get into accidents, or who, I believe, end up with Parkinson's disease, and so forth. I think if you see these people early on, there is a death wish that causes their condition. You know, they don't want to live. They don't want to look at this. They don't want to look at that."

Finally, like many of the others quoted here, he believes that one of the most healing aspects of relationships is that they can help us bear and express our feelings. "My point is that when somebody is in a loving relationship or grows up in a loving family, that person's ability to tolerate painful feelings goes up dramatically. When you don't have love in your life, your ability to tolerate, endure, and experience painful feelings goes down. So people who don't have love in their lives don't have the nurturing, the softness, the comfort, the insulation to be able to experience painful feelings. When they come home, instead of being able to feel what they feel, share it with someone and let go of it, they drown their sorrows with alcohol, with addictive behaviors. Exercise is good, but people can overexercise and die. They use exercise as a way of altering their mood, their hormones, so that they cannot feel their connection with the world, they cannot feel their emptiness and loneliness. Without love in your life, a healthy person will become depressed. But this is a healthy depression, motivating you to fill that void. If you have all kinds of substitutes to prevent you from feeling your loneliness — like overexercising, watching too much television, overdrinking, oversleeping — those things will cause you to be out of touch with your feelings. If you don't do these things, what you'll feel is the pain of not having love. And then you will be motivated to get out of pain. Avoidance of pain is the greatest motivator that exists.

"A loving relationship, for example, allows us to stay in touch with our day-to-day feelings of what is going on. We have someone to come home to, share, talk, connect with. So we don't have to suppress the uncomfortable feelings of the day, we don't need to be dependent upon drugs and alcohol to run away from those uncomfortable feelings. Instead, you come home to someone who loves you. That love, it draws those feelings out. It makes those uncomfortable feelings bearable, so you can feel them, and hear them, and let go of them. Without love, those feelings can't come out. . . . To the extent that we are disconnected from the source of life, from who we are, our ability to *feel* becomes restricted. It's by being in touch with our feelings and feeling loved that we are able to heal ourselves."

Candace B. Pert, Ph.D., is research professor in the department of physiology and biophysics at Georgetown University Medical Center in Washington, D.C., where she also conducts AIDS research. She was a discoverer of the opiate receptor. She is the author of the book *Molecules of Emotion: Why We Feel the Way We Feel.*

Dr. Pert has an extraordinary point of view: Love and intimacy clearly affect our health and survival, but not because the mind affects the body. According to her, there is no fundamental distinction between the mind and the body. "I call this system the *bodymind,* because in it, the emotions are inextricably linked with our physiology. The mind, the emotions, are not just in the brain. It doesn't all stop at the neck."

In her view, the cells themselves are intimate with each other. "Virtually every cell in the body is sensing something. Why? Because we're not composed of little, disconnected test tubes of cells, even though that is how scientists like to break it all down to study things. The living cells in humans are quite different. Each cell has to be in communication with the rest of the cells in the body to make one integrated whole. So the actual purpose of our emotions, as carried by these biochemicals, these peptides, is to keep us operating as an integrated whole." In other words, intimacy is healing even at a cellular level!

I said that it seemed like she was describing a mechanism to explain how emotions affect us, even at a cellular level.

"Yes. And they do. They affect us even at a cellular level and also run every system in our bodies. . . . The research I've been involved in for the last twenty years suggests that our emotions are intertwined with every aspect of our physiology. People in the conventional medical paradigm are currently talking about serotonin and neurons, and little tiny control centers for the emotions in the brain. But, in fact, the emotions originate as a field that flows all around and through the brain, glands, immune system, heart, and intestines, making up a complete informational network. So, the first thing is to not think about emotions as being isolated in the brain, and this gives us a paradigm for seeing how emotional health or emotional disease could impact on every aspect of our physiology.

"There are over a hundred different substances in the organism which we call *informational substances*. Many, but not all, are peptides — short strings of amino acids — that act at receptors on the surface of cells all over the body."

I asked why she thinks emotions like loneliness, depression, cynicism, hostility, and isolation have such toxic effects.

"I have this notion that bliss is hardwired when we are in intimate, loving relationships. The reason negative emotions such as loneliness or cynicism have such toxic effects is that they are not normal, natural states. Our ancestors didn't have them, or they would have died out without passing their genes on — they never would have mated. I believe we are hardwired to feel good and to have good, strong relationships. But our culture is very disruptive of that. People used to be very tight and depended on their friends and families. Now, we are in this very different era, where people fly across the country, and so can be alone quite a lot. I don't think those states are natural. I don't think they are normal.

"We are mammals, which is really critical. We do not have thousands of young, and, randomly, five of them live. We have only a few, and we are very bonded to our children, to our spouses. I think we have that inclination built right into our bodymind structure. We were set up so that we could survive, and we have these chemicals to help us. We are programmed to have strong human relationships, and that is how we evolved, from bands of people who had these kinds of bonds. So the people who survive today are the ones whose ancestors did well communicating, were in loving relationships with others, with their extended families. People today may ignore that and think they can go off without it, but we are stuck with the same bodyminds, the same chemistry, that our ancestors had."

I asked her to describe some of the mechanisms that connect our emotions and our cells.

"I go back to health, to wholeness and integrity, and the body operating without overstressing, the way it was intended to operate. Take cancer, for example. We have mechanisms to destroy tumors that grow naturally in the body every day. Natural killer cells, part of our immune system, actually have receptors, and they squirt out peptides which are identical to the molecules of emotion. The cancer cells themselves are actually squirting peptides and also being modulated by peptide receptors on their surface, telling them to divide or not divide, to metastasize or not metastasize. Since the tumors are part of our bodies, they are also in the psycho-somatic network, the information flow. All of this is very much governed by our emotional state, our emotional molecules. There are many experiments to show how these tumor cells are being modulated by various growth factors, endorphins, peptides, and substances which are found in the brain and the immune system.

"So our immune systems do reflect our state of mind, our emotions. The immune system is important, not just in cancer, but for fighting off viruses. If we are not in an integrated, healthy home, being fed by the nurturing relationships that our bodies were designed to have, I think the immune system breaks down. It gets overactive, resulting in autoimmune disease, or it gets underactive, producing cancers. It just doesn't seem surprising to me at all that this happens."

Dr. Pert believes that it is a false distinction to separate our emotions and our immune system.

"They *are* our emotional states. The question really is: Do the molecules cause the emotion, or do the emotions cause the release of the molecules? It gets close to the secret of life. The emotions actually modulate the mechanisms in our immune system that create our very body fabric. If you cut or burn yourself, within seconds new cells, immune cells, arrive at the site to rebuild and heal the injury. They squirt out peptides and orchestrate a whole well-coordinated repair mechanism. Our healing mechanisms are truly governed by these emotions, and it can all shut down."

"Some studies," I said, "have shown that if you infect people with a cold virus, the ones who actually develop a cold are those with the fewest social contacts when compared to the others."

"That's interesting, because we now know, from research done over the past ten years, that virtually all viruses use receptors on the cell surface to get into cells. And they can't get into any cell. Each virus has a protein envelope surrounding its surface that is tailor-made to allow the virus to latch onto and enter specific cells, thereby infecting them. These receptors are the identical receptors that I have been talking about in the psychosomatic network, many of which are associated with emotional tones. So, depending on how much natural chemical one has on board, how much natural ligand there is to bind and fit into specified receptors, those cells can be occupied, or blocked, by the natural substance, preventing the virus from entering. The virus which causes colds is actually known to use the norepinephrine receptor. Norepinephrine has been associated with excitement, with anticipating pleasure. People who are bummed out, I would imagine, have less of that substance circulating around their systems, and that leaves an empty receptor through which the virus can enter the cell and infect it. I am speculating this could be the emotional mechanism that is the link, right there."

I asked her why altruism may enhance immune function.

"Having loving relationships is how we evolved. The people who didn't have the mechanisms for this died out millions of years ago, but we have them, and it puts us in the right frame of bodymind for healing and survival to occur. E. O. Wilson, the famous biologist, actually talked about how there had to be a biological basis for altruism, or it wouldn't continue to exist. The people who have survived today are the people who have these things. If you deny this and go against the natural way our bodyminds are wired, you may get away with it for a little while. We do have the power to subvert what is going on in our bodies, to be in our heads, and not be loving or connected, but it has a cost. Eventually, our natural chemicals, our molecules of emotion, become suppressed and don't go where they should go, and I think that is what truly leads to diseased states."

Redford B. Williams, Jr., M.D., is Professor and Director of the Behavioral Medicine Research Center at Duke University Medical Center. His important research studies have clearly documented the role of hostility in premature death and disease. He is the author of several books, including *Anger Kills*.

Dr. Williams, like Dr. Syme, is interested in the relation of social support to socioeconomic status. "These various psychosocial risk factors — hostility, social isolation or support, depression, anxiety, even high job strain — don't occur in isolation from one another; they tend to co-occur in the same people. They are by no means one to one, but they are strongly associated. Also, they tend to cluster in low-socioeconomic-status people even more, and may, indeed, account for some of the excess of premature mortality that poor people have. As you go down in socioeconomic status, hostility, depression, and job strain go up, and social support goes down.

"Along with hostility — as well as depression and social isolation — is a set of behaviors and biological characteristics. The behaviors are more drinking, more smoking, more eating. Hostile people consume six hundred more calories a day, on average, than those with low hostility. I think this is because of low serotonin. While eating a meal, there is an increase in serotonin release. It may very well be the case that eating is a way of medicating yourself with serotonin, causing it to release in certain parts of the brain and calm you down and calm down an overactive sympathetic nervous system.

"But from any of these things — the smoking, the eating, the alcohol use, the overactive sympathetic nervous system — you don't go directly to disease. I think it has to go through molecular and cellular mechanisms. Here's where my scientific bias comes out, but I think that ultimately, if you are talking about disease processes like failure to reject tumors or accelerated development of atherogenic plaques, you have got to talk about things that affect the cellular and molecular processes that are directly involved. That is why we are looking at the immune system, stress hormones like catecholamines and cortisol, the stress-induced stimulation of the sympathetic nervous system, and the lack of parasympathetic antagonism of those effects. And the smoking, the eating, and the higher cholesterol all play into this."

I asked why we would evolve in a way that is so clearly destructive, that goes against our survival.

"There may be an evolutionary advantage to having a pretty robust sympathetic nervous system activation that doesn't get turned off so fast by the parasympathetic, if all you've got to do is survive long enough to father or mother some children. Indeed, that may have been critical for survival at some point. When you consider the literally millions of years it took for those mechanisms to evolve, it's only been probably within the last ten thousand years that the necessity for those kinds of reactions has been shrinking. You don't need a fight-or-flight response in traffic or in a supermarket line, or when you are trying to get your teenage son to clean up his room. So these reactions become maladaptive."

"Take off your scientific hat for a moment," I asked. "You did a study at Duke University with 1,400 men and women who underwent coronary angiography and had at least one severely blocked artery. After five years, men and women who were unmarried and who did not have a close confidant — someone to talk with on a regular basis — were over *three times* as likely to have died than those who were married, had a confidant, or both. Why do you think that is? It goes beyond molecules, don't you think?"

"No. I don't. I think, ultimately, everything will have to come down to molecules. I think in the Duke study, something about being that isolated had effects on their behavior and on their biology in ways that precipitated earlier mortality — whether directly through arrhythmias, or indirectly through a more rapid progression of their atherosclerotic process. People don't just drop dead without something going on at the cellular-molecular levels."

He described a number of biological mechanisms by which a lack of love and an excess of hostility might lead to disease and premature death. These included an overactive sympathetic nervous system, which can lead to electrical instability and cardiac arrhythmias; hormones such as epinephrine and norepinephrine (adrenaline); changes in immune function; atherosclerosis; changes in beta receptors; and so on. "I think for sudden death, it can be electrical instability. Jim Mueller, at the University of Kentucky, did a study which showed that during the two hours following an episode of intense anger, your risk of having a heart attack is doubled. But that doesn't mean we can't do something about it.

"I have a classic hostile personality type. I'm one of these people I talk about. It took my wife Virginia telling me, 'I'm not going to keep on putting up with the way you are treating me,' along with what I was finding in my research, to motivate me to change. I'm a lot better than I used to be, but when I get tired or jet-lagged or something — boy, you wouldn't believe some of the crazy things I can do."

I was curious to know what he did when he found himself doing the very things that he knows are so harmful.

"I ask myself, 'Is this really that important? Is it really appropriate for me to be getting upset with this little old lady who is driving ahead of me? Is this a situation that I can really expect to change?' And if I get a *no* to any of those things, I try to chill out. Or if I get a *yes* to all of them, I ask myself one last question: 'Is it worth it to invest the energy to change it?' Actually, sometimes it is, and then I act. Most of the time, it isn't."

I asked, "Do you believe that with enough scientific studies, we will find the mechanistic explanations for why loneliness, isolation, depression, and hostility affect us to such a degree?"

"Yes. I think, ultimately, everything will have to come down to molecules. As Lord Kelvin once said, 'When you can assign numbers to something, you are on your way to really understanding it.' We used to ascribe the movement of the sun to a god driving a chariot across the sky every day."

"But people could chart the course of the sun before they necessarily knew the mechanisms behind its movement," I said.

When I asked him why a lack of love and intimacy might cause changes in molecules and mechanisms, he replied, "If we don't get enough of the normal nurturing as children, our brain serotonin systems don't develop normally. We grow up to have a brain that is more likely to be sensitive to forces that cause it to be depressed, hostile, and socially isolated, as well as having the biological and behavioral characteristics that predispose to disease. My reasoning is, then, that the lack of nurturing from one's parents in childhood affects these biological processes in ways that set all of this in motion. So, yes, love — it's the lack of love that really causes it."

"But, clearly, you don't think it's all just serotonin?"

"That is one way I can *biologically* explain it. It's not the only way, and in fact, an equally important path is that just living in a harsh, unloving environment can teach you that the world is a hostile place, is a depressing place. It can cause you to have — just from the stress of that environment — an overactive sympathetic nervous system."

He ended on a hopeful note: "If we could teach people how to deal with the negative emotions which seem to be keeping them from realizing the potential that love might have to offer, then love might have a better chance to grow and heal, not only ourselves, but those we love."

James H. Billings, Ph.D., M.P.H., has degrees in clinical psychology, epidemiology, and divinity — an interesting combination. We have collaborated on several research studies over the past thirteen years. I asked Dr. Billings to describe, from his various perspectives, the shift from the psychology of the group to that of the individual.

"I'm fifty-four years old. And my genes are — let's just say for easy math — one million years old. If I think about it, all I needed was one relative to get eaten before they procreated somewhere along the forty millionth combination and permutation of those genes, and I wouldn't have been born. So, everything had to go right, for a long time, for me to be here.

"For centuries, one of the things that a child had to learn to do to survive was to understand the expectations, the norm, of the clan or the tribe and, with relatively little conflict, to obey them. Because if they did the wrong thing at the wrong time, if they made a noise at the wrong time, if they decided to act out at the wrong time, it's not just that the child might die, but also the larger group might not survive, either. So part of what children were born with was a capacity to inhibit themselves in order to meet the expectations of the normative group or the clan that they belonged to.

"The picture is then complicated by the advent of participatory democracies, which is only about four thousand years ago. At that point, the relative role and the nature of man began to get redefined, so that the individual became more and more important. This movement was relatively small in the beginning and gained momentum in the early 1600s. It was the beginning of a change in the definition of a person as a member of a tribe or group to a unique individual with specific social responsibilities, including an individual relationship with God. This is part of what the Reformation was about: the belief that an individual no longer needed the intercession of the church to have a relationship with God.

"Western psychology, which is a little more than one hundred years old, really redefined man by developing a new paradigm of what is normal and what is abnormal. The focus shifted almost completely to the individual. The very idea that someone was dependent on another person was diagnostic of any number of pathologies. These people were usually the ones who were often depressed, who were feeling isolated, abandoned, and they were having a hard time getting someone to respond to their condition.

"In my dissertation, I followed a group of people for five years after they were hospitalized for attempting suicide. The notion at that time was that people who were in psychotherapy would be better off than people who were not in treatment. I was surprised to find that the people in therapy were killing themselves at a substantially higher rate than the others! I was trying to understand what was going on. What came up, over and over again, was that the people killing themselves in treatment were seeing an analytic therapist who maintained a detached distance from them — they would lie on a couch, not able to see the therapist, who would say very little to the patient during a session. The patient was having an enormous need to make contact with the therapist and to have him or her respond in a nurturing, caring way; when the therapist didn't, the patient often ended up attempting suicide or actually killing himself or herself. Nowadays, a therapist does not stay in a detached mode when a patient is suicidal and now recognizes that maintaining a distance is going to make the person worse.

"So we have a world full of people who have a genetic predisposition to affiliation, the need to belong, and we still have a psychological development theory that defines what is normal as making sure that people are not dependent in their relationships. It says that affiliation is pathological, that what you really need to be healthy is to not need anybody. These psychological constructs define what is normal in ways that are at odds with our biology, that thwart affiliation and add to the demise of the family. This approach is defining child-rearing practices, relationships with children, and relationships with spouses."

He then described how this shift in Western psychology has intensified the isolation of the individual from the group, and how this threatens our survival. "There has been a very powerful notion in psychotherapy that if anything is wrong with a child, it's the parents' fault — they are to blame. People who grow up in that kind of system become parents themselves and are terrified to do anything, because they're afraid of doing something wrong. As a result, children are left with a lack of clear guidelines about social norms. Our survival response tells us if we violate the social norm then we'll get kicked out of the tribe, but since we don't know what the norm is, we never know what we're supposed to do. We are frightened of making a mistake, frightened of being found out. Everybody then is operating within the same basic system, which is try to look like everybody else, try to behave like everybody else, so nobody gets found out that they don't belong — even though they don't feel like they belong in the first place!"

I replied, "Our group support sessions give people a safe place where they can talk about and find out that other people often struggle with the same issues and feelings."

"Exactly. In some cases, they're not even big things; they just happen to be feelings that people in our culture usually don't share, so we assume we are the only ones who feel this way. In that way, we are isolated. As soon as people are talking about shared experiences, they realize that they are not so different. Whatever you are struggling with — your fears, your worries — you are sharing your life in real time as you go along with a group of people. It has become a community with which you share the common experience of your life. It's part of the appeal of your books because you talk about your own feelings and vulnerability.

"It resonates to the tribal experience of 100,000 years ago when people did everything together. There were no secrets. Everybody knew everything about everybody, yet people were still there for you. The very definition of the tribe included you. The bad thing was you were stuck in that role."

I asked him why he thinks these factors affect disease and mortality to such a strong degree.

"Because we are in a state of arousal all the time if we don't have them. Biologically, we need a place where we belong, a place where we are seen, we are visible, we feel welcome, a place where we can talk easily and we can listen easily. Most people spend their entire life feeling apprehensive, not feeling like they belong anyplace. The world doesn't provide this for us. The institutions in which we normally had a sense of community are eroding. Also, we have the impact of modern technology — airplanes, trains, cars. One hundred and fifty years ago, families stayed intact because they lived in proximity to one another. That is very unusual now."

I asked, "Weren't you glad to grow up and leave your family?"

"Yes, but I realize I lost something profound when I moved away. Even in its craziness, I had a place there. Now, I have friends, a family, people who form a community we have chosen. It's a group of people who we are connected to because they want that connection as much as we do. There are lots of people out there who have relationships, but they're tense and anxious, on their best behavior, trying to look good, to act right. There's still no place where they are seen, where they belong, no place where they can just flop, relax, and be themselves. There is nothing to provide a buffer. If I am stressed at work and I have nothing to go home to that is comforting, I can't deal with the stress. I can deal with stress or demands there if I am safe here. But what happens for many people is that there is no place that is safe. They go home and sit in front of the TV and try to go into a trance state. They essentially hibernate. They go from arousal to a kind of trance state."

Like Dr. Berkman, he feels strongly about the need to become embedded in the social fabric. The concept of duty to the tribe or family is not an onerous thing but something we can pursue willingly and even joyfully.

"Absolutely. It's a definition. It's a role. It's a part of who I am. *Our biology requires affiliation.* In general, it's not what you are getting; it's how you serve the tribe. The world is oriented to *self.* I'm not saying you never make a selfish choice. But, at this particular point, we've gone from 'There is nothing but duty' to 'There is nothing but self.' And there has to be something in between. We are out of control at this point, and trying to find our way back to a balanced life. It's all about finding the balance."

Harvey Zarren, M.D., is a board-certified cardiologist and Associate Clinical Professor of Medicine at the Tufts University School of Medicine in Boston. He practices medicine in Lynn, Massachusetts, a blue-collar community, where he is director of the cardiac rehabilitation program.

"Virtually every coronary patient that I see, even in the coronary care unit, I ask, 'With whom do you share your feelings?'

They look at me like I'm from outer space. 'What's that got to do with my heart?' It's also a good opening for helping people to understand how much their mind and their feelings are associated with their heart.

"The men always say they don't share their feelings with anyone, and the women say that they share the good stuff with their daughter or someone but they don't want to burden anybody with what's really bothering them. I ask them to find someone in their life — anyone — with whom they can sit down and tell that person, 'The doctor says I have to share my feelings a little bit every day, and when I do, you are not to give me any advice or judgment unless I ask.' Because if you constantly get judged, you don't want to share. If they constantly are having to come up with answers, they really don't want to listen after a while. You tell that person, 'If you do it for me, I'll do it for you.' Men, surprisingly, say to me, 'Doc, I'm telling George in the shop stuff I haven't told anybody in years, and I really don't care so much now.'

"When people begin to be real with their feelings, things happen in their bodies' physiology that encourage healing. It's just amazing to watch. I think our knowledge of how that happens is so superficial.

"I have one personal experience of a former neighbor of mine who had pancreatic cancer who called me up. I spent three hours a week with her for nine months. Her disease was so extensive, she was told she was going to be dead in six months. She went to see a surgeon at the Mass General Hospital; he looked at her CT scan [X ray] and he said, 'This visit is a waste of my time and your time. You are going to be dead shortly, and nothing will help.'

"That's when she called me. She went through an incredible transformation over nine months. I spent a lot of time with her, and it was just incredible. She was cross-country skiing. When she had a second CT scan six months later, the radiologist said to me that they must have mislabeled it because the tumor had shrunk. Before, she had tumor mass everywhere, and it really shrank. She was also getting 5-FU as chemotherapy, but that doesn't do much; I don't think that accounted for her improvement.

"When it became clear that she wasn't going to cure this cancer, I changed the kind of work I was doing with her. She came up with a meditation that allayed her fear of dying, and then it reduced *my* fear of *her* dying. It was a picture of her going down a meadow with a butterfly on her finger and a bird on her shoulder and then just becoming one with the sunlight, and it just kind of . . . it changed both of us forever. She ended up dying nine months later, but with this amazing, amazing capacity to be real for the first time in her life.

"The thing that frustrates me the most is every time I see another article where they are trying to isolate a molecule so they can make a pill so people don't have to do the emotional work. It's just as you said — it's about avoiding being real. Every time they come up with something that allows people to behave the old, unreal, closed-in way, and somehow take a pill so that they don't have to take responsibility for their own growth and development, it just seems counterproductive to me."

I asked him to speculate on why medicine evolved this way.

"I think that the average physician comes out of a background based on two historical events. The first was the Flexner Report in 1910. That report talked about science and mathematics and physics but said nothing in it about people. It had a profound effect on medical education in this country. The second was the advent of antibiotics. Before that, if you had pneumococcal pneumonia, you had to believe you were going to get well to have a 50 percent chance, probably, of surviving. Once penicillin came around, they just gave you penicillin. No one cared what you believed, and they didn't care what they said at the bedside anymore. I think those two events have created a medical education that has such enormous tunnel vision because it is based on feedback from a technologically and economically based society that drives medical education and leaves caregivers blind. They are blind to being human; they are blind to the effect of humanity on health. They are clearly blind to nutrition."

I asked him how this has affected how he now teaches medicine.

"I run a course now at Tufts — a one-month rotation called *Cardiology as a Healing Art*. I did it because of a medical student who came to me in her third year and said, "I want to study with you, but I don't want to study cardiology. I want to study healing." I dropped my cardiology rotation, and the school supported this. I have these extraordinary students who come out so thirsty just to sit at a bedside and talk to a human being. I started to build a curriculum, and it just turns out that every student is so different."

"What do you do?"

"Well, one of the things that I do is I have a student spend a day with a nurse. I say, 'I want you to look at the color of her skin, her aura, her facial expression, how she emotes, and what she says every time during the day she has contact with the physician.' It's amazing. They come back and say, 'What are we doing to these people? We're torturing them!' I say, 'Well, you remember. You are going to be on the other end of that phone one day.' And I have them go through the hospitals seeing how different people behave when they respond to doctors. It's pathetic. We'll go on rounds in the morning. The first patient I come to, I'll say, 'Sit with this lady and find out what she really thinks about being in our hospital. Tell her that it's not going to be told to anybody else, and you can have as much time as you want. Call me when you're done. If it takes all day, it's fine. If it takes two days, that's fine. No time limit.' They suddenly find out they are talking to human beings. The patients fall in love with them. I take them to funerals. I take them to wakes. I'll sit in the stairs and cry with them when somebody dies. I'll take them to a cardiac arrest, and then go read twenty-five EKGs, do three stress tests, go back, read another sixty EKGs and then run to the emergency room, and then show them how there is no time in the course of a day to emotionally process anything. At the end of a day, I'm left angry, and you know where that goes — it goes home."

"I admire what you are doing," I said. "Take off your conventional cardiology hat for a moment, and speculate why you think loneliness and isolation and depression and anger are linked so strongly with premature death and disease from virtually all causes?"

"I think human beings are looking for love and connection. We are intrinsically social organisms, and I think we are living in a culture that does not understand wellness in any sense of the word, a culture that only understands money. What happens is that people starve; it's an impoverishment of self. It's like someone who has no white cells. You can dump antibiotics in them forever and they will still die of infection. I tell all my cardiac patients, 'If you are tired, I don't think it's necessarily the disease. It's struggling to be well in a culture that doesn't understand wellness.' I really believe that a lot of what we see as disease states, as altered immune systems or however it's manifested, is a starvation for love and connection. I really believe that. Our knowledge of the mechanisms is incredibly superficial."

I added that many businesses are beginning to see the importance of these ideas even from a business perspective.

"Yes — I spoke at the annual meeting of the American Society of Health Risk Managers a year ago. They asked, 'What is the risk of bringing alternative therapies into hospitals?' I said, 'The risk is if you don't do it, your hospital is going to be left behind. That's a big risk. But the other big risk is a personal one. With the exception of maybe acupuncture, most of the alternative therapies require you to open up as a human being, and a lot of people find that risky.'

"I started a program at our hospital called *The Healing Connection*. This is something that the hospital just took on as its corporate identity. The vision statement says, 'We will put people and the value of human interaction back into the center of healing.' We now have two business consultants pushing this through all fifteen hundred people in the hospital. Somebody from senior management said, 'What are you talking about? What is this?' I said, 'Patients want to be touched, they want to be loved, and they want to be hugged. They want to be heard.' He said, 'You've got to teach us about this.' So, I did a workshop for senior management. You know what I found out? They want to be touched and they want to be heard. So, then the board of trustees wanted to know what the workshop was about, so I did a workshop for them, and I found out that *they* wanted to be touched and heard and loved. We were able to talk about that through the institution.

"I said to them, 'You know, there is no difference between that poor Spanish lady coming in with pneumonia and you and the board. You are both human beings. You may have more money than she does, but you've got the same troubles at home.'"

I responded, "Well, that is the essence of compassion, which to me is the essence of healing — when people make that recognition."

"It's an absolute necessity for people to be connected and to be cared for and to be cared about. I think it's just *real*. It's unfortunate that some people continue to get wrapped up in the *why*. In programs for reversing heart disease, it is the group interaction that is the most important factor, not just diet."

"And yet it's the one that is often least valued," I replied. "When I present our research findings at a scientific meeting, the other scientists often say, 'Yes, we believe your data and we now believe that heart disease is reversible. But, of course, it's all due to your diet and exercise, and this touchy-feely stuff has no bearing whatsoever except maybe to the extent that it helps people stay on the diet and exercise better.' "

"See, I think it's the other way around. I think the touchy-feely stuff is the stuff that works. I really do."

I mentioned that some people believe that this is an upper-middle-class phenomenon, and lower socioeconomic groups really aren't interested in these kinds of issues.

"Oh, absolutely the reverse. I think these people find it easier. They're not caught up in all the nonsense. When people are not quite as educated, if you can show them something that works, that feels good, then they grab it. They don't torture themselves with mind games. If you can take a lady who has got a high school education, six kids, who is smoking and has a heart attack at age forty-two, and you can show her that she can go into a group, be listened to, and people will care about her, then she will come every week. And she will do better, and she will stay on the diet. She doesn't torture herself with reading philosophy and randomized controlled trials and people bending her this way and that. She's got nothing out there, and if she can find something that helps her, she'll stick to it."

"That has also been my experience," I agreed.

Daniel Goleman, Ph.D., has been a science correspondent for the *New York Times* for many years, focusing on issues related to psychology and behavior. He is also the author of several books, including *Emotional Intelligence.*

I asked Dr. Goleman to explain why love and intimacy are such important factors in health and well-being. "There are two potent and relevant concepts in this data. One is that emotions are contagious, and the second is that our tool kit for managing our own emotions involves other people to a very great extent. Elaine Hatfield wrote a book about this called *Emotional Contagion.* In relationships, people are continually making other people feel better — that is, managing anxiety, getting someone out of being sad, dealing with anger — or worse. And people are doing this in the natural course of things, not with any specific intent. Just as when you are in a bad mood, one of the things you can do is get together with someone who will make you feel better. If you don't have people in your life who can do that, and if your own internal armamentarium isn't that effective for it, then you are stuck in a toxic state."

I asked him to identify what mechanisms that might explain, even in part, why love and intimacy have such powerful effects across cultures, across species, across socio-economic groups, across disease states.

"The emotional centers of the brain have some of the heaviest networks going out of the brain into the immune system, into the gut, and into the cardiovascular system. Did you know there are neurons for empathy located in the brain? There may be a system, at a profound neurological level, designed to enfold both the individual immune system and the social encounter. I think it may have coevolved that way. Systems almost always evolve in ways that have the most survival value. Our brain is designed to be part of a social system. There's a theory that the neo-cortex — and, actually, large parts of the cortex — evolved in order to keep track of social groups. The larger the primate band, the larger the cortex found in primates. The new, more positive look at Darwinism is that the survival of the fittest means the survival of the most fecund — the ones who have the most children are the ones that survive, and the way to do that is by cooperating. So there is a very large evolutionary pressure for mechanisms that foster cooperation and co-hesion. I suspect that may have coevolved with the linkup of the neurologic and the immune systems in humans, probably even before humans, since it's in the mammalian brain as well."

I pointed out that there is also a strong tendency toward selfishness, isolation, and individualism in our society.

"I don't believe it is equally as strong. I think if it were equally as strong, there would be far fewer people on the planet. I think the John Wayne, every-man-for-himself individuality in our culture is an aberration in evolution. For example, if you observe the way primates are, they really hang together. A socially isolated lifestyle is not something you find in the primate world much at all. Isolation does occur in nature, but primates who are selfish tend to be social rejects. The same is true for humans: If you don't share, if you don't cooperate, then people don't like you very much. I think we started getting out of whack with the rise of civilization, when we stopped being dependent on small bands for our mutual survival. At that point, we started to have what amounts to *social mutations in our behavior* — mutations that weren't so dysfunctional that people who pursued such courses would actually perish."

I asked, "What contribution do you think modern psychology and Freud made with their emphasis on the individual, often at the expense of the family, sometimes even blaming the family?"

"I don't place the emphasis on the individual at the foot of the psychologists. I see it differently. Many, if not most, cultures in the world actually have a huge emphasis on group identity, rather than on an individual identity — like Japan, China, and most tribal groups everywhere. The idea of an individual self is something that arose largely with European Renaissance thinking, or post-Renaissance, during the Enlightenment. The individualist orientation arose with the bourgeois, and with mercantilism, as a philosophical stance and a cultural stance in Europe. It spread to America and was taken up very much by Americans because of the sense of ego in the American society. It has been superimposed on other societies with the spread of Western ways, but it's a foreign concept in most parts of the world. It spread to America, perhaps, because the people who came here were, in one sense, renegades and loners."

"But even then, it was 'We the people.' "

"Yes, it was. In fact, people needed community to survive here very much in the early days. The individualist character is a frontier phenomenon. Harry Triandis talks about the differences between individualist and collectivist cultures. Collectivist cultures are very enmeshed. People count on each other, depend on each other. Social emotions are very prominent, such as embarrassment and shame, in those cultures, as regulatory mechanisms."

"You have written extensively on meditation and other spiritual practices, and you are close with the Dalai Lama. My working thesis is that anything that creates a sense of connectedness is healing, whether it's with other people, or with split-off parts of yourself, or with a higher power — God, the experience of interconnectedness, the one Self. How would you describe that?"

"That's very interesting. The Buddhist understanding of what it means to be empty — a word often mis-translated — is clinging to the notion that you are only a separate self. The dialogue about this, which I love, is that emptiness is really very full, very rich. You develop a lightness of being when you're not so attached or clinging to a strong ego identity, and you experience much more directly the rich interrelatedness of the web you actually exist in. In other words, you experience connectedness. It's a state of union."

James S. House, Ph.D., is Director of the Survey Research Center and Professor of Sociology at the University of Michigan in Ann Arbor. He was the director of the Tecumseh Community Health Study. Dr. House offered his perspective on why social support is such a powerful phenomenon.

"We did a review article in the journal *Science* about three major kinds of mechanisms, which I still think are probably ones that count for a good deal of the effect. These mechanisms are all interrelated.

"The most obvious one is the sense of support — having people who can help or support people emotionally, instrumentally, tangibly, and otherwise, when they have problems. People seem to derive a good deal of benefit from feeling they have — or *perceiving* they have — supportive relationships with other people. There are potential benefits that don't necessarily require actual support being delivered in any direct way. It seems to be more that feeling that one has someone, somewhere, whom one can turn to. Simply *believing* one has support can be beneficial, independent of whether it actually occurs or not.

"The two others we talk about in the article are probably equally important in different ways. One is the sense that other people provide a kind of social control over people's lives and behaviors. This is one that's often missed, and I think it's one that may help account for why the presence and existence of relationships are somewhat independent of their quality. There are people who will maintain relationships that are highly damaging. Most people try to choose relationships, as best they can, that are at least mutual. But something like marriage — one finds a beneficial effect of people being married, or having some comparable relationship, that seems to be somewhat independent of the type of qualities of that relationship. When someone is married, they have someone present to monitor their behavior — and they are more likely to monitor their own — smoking, eating, drinking, exercise, risky behavior, and so on.

"The third point is a sense that people need people. Or, even more generally, mammals need other mammals, in some basic biological sense, or, conceivably, spiritual sense as well. There seem to be calming effects from the mere presence of other people, mediated via a range of physiological processes and mechanisms. Negative relationships can have the opposite effect on people, but, across a fairly broad band of relationships, there seem to be positive effects of people having other people in contact with them when they are going through stressful circumstances."

I asked him if all of it can be reduced to biological mechanisms.

"No, probably not. There is a tendency to think, ultimately, many of the mechanisms have to be physiological in nature — biochemical, or endocrine, or whatever. Clearly, not all of them are. I think we have to look at some of the mechanisms that are more purely social and psychological in nature. For example, the mechanisms that involve control of behavior, or regulation or influence on behavior, really operate at a more behavioral level. If someone stops or reduces smoking in response to another person, and somebody avoids taking risks or engages in safer behaviors, like using seat belts, the protective mechanism doesn't require going beyond that. You could say that, obviously, what is being avoided by wearing your seat belt is that you don't get thrown against the windshield, and you don't have trauma — but that is sort of elaborating what might happen. I think there is a real mechanism there, that is at the more behavioral level of what makes a person decide to wear a seat belt in the first place."

I asked, "Why, then, is just the belief that someone cares about you so beneficial, whether or not it affects your behavior?"

"One of the characteristics of social support, as well as some other psychosocial factors, is they seem to have these rather broad and pervasive effects on physiological functioning, so you don't necessarily find highly cause-specific or disease-specific effects. Instead, you find the rather phenomenally large effects that you are talking about on all-cause mortality, or on overall health. Depending on what the individual's other risk factors are or what other threats or insults are in their environment, they may benefit — some in one way, some through a different mechanism. For example, social support causes changes in immune system that tend to make people more resistant to infectious diseases, possibly even more resistant to progression of cancers or tumors. These psychosocial factors may be mediated via central nervous system and neuroendocrine pathways that seem to control or modulate cardiac activity, blood pressure, and heart rate. Also, I think there is evidence of mechanisms of reduction in the production of fatty acids, which are cholesterol-type substances in the blood stream. There are all kinds of effects going on, only some of which we can measure."

I replied, "In science, as you know, people are always looking for objective, reproducible measures. If you simply count the number of relationships, it's easier for someone else to reproduce your findings. If you talk about perception of experience, it is, by definition, harder to reproduce yet perhaps more meaningful."

"The crude indicators, which often have been used in long-term longitudinal studies, are these: Are you married? How often do you see or talk to other people? Do you go to church? Do you participate in other organizations? Those are simply proxies for a set of relationships or interactions that people have. Many scientists have the impression that what the observer can see or measure is, in some ways, more real, more valid, important, reliable, than that which a person can report to us. I just don't think that is true. Certainly, there are errors and biases in what people report and tell us, but I think that there are also errors in measurement by blood pressure instruments and all kinds of observer ratings."

I commented that in this context, the term *social support* doesn't quite do it justice. It seemed that we were really talking about love and intimacy, even though those words, like religion, tend to frighten off many scientists.

"I think that all of these things are important. Clearly, love and intimacy are perhaps the highest forms of social release and supported, even in certain kinds of spiritual relationships. But we ought not to exaggerate the extent to which a relationship has to have all of these ideals and qualities in order for it to be helpful and beneficial to people. I think that people benefit in terms of health in a variety of other ways, from a range of relationships that may not be ones we would qualify or quantify as being highly intimate, highly loving relationships — but they are still positive and beneficial relationships.

"I think there is a variety of evidence for humans, and across a range of species, that says we are basically organisms that need relationships with other people in order to grow, develop, maintain, and sustain ourselves in a variety of ways. You can explain this either spiritually or in an evolutionary way, if you want. We need these relationships, in a whole range of ways, some of which are more tangible than others. We need other people to be able to satisfy our physical needs, but we also need other people to satisfy our emotional or analytical needs. There is a sense, whether you take it from religion or psychology, that people have a need for meaning, coherence, understanding of the world. People need a sense that their life, their existence, has some purpose, and, for many people, that sense of meaning and purpose is defined most proximately, and probably most strongly, by the relationships they have with other people — with spouses; with other family, parents, children; with friends; with people they associate with at work or in voluntary organizations.

"When you look at something like religion, it's another area that has been less explored (because I think the scientific community tends to be a relatively areligious one, on the whole). What we know suggests that there may well be health benefits of religion. That is one component of most of the social integration types of measures that have been used in mortality studies, looking at things like frequency in church attendance or involvement in religious activities. I don't think we know fully what it is people are getting, whether it's a theological sense of meaning, or whether it's the elements of regulation of behavior within religious groups — more extreme in some than the others. For example, Mormons and Seventh-Day Adventists have lifestyles that are very different because of their religion. Also, you have the social contacts, relationships, and activities that go along with involvement in religious activities and the sense of purpose that people derive from these. So, there is a range of possibilities."

I asked how much influence Western psychology has had on the emphasis of the individual at the expense of the community.

"I don't think we ought to lay it all on the doorstep of anybody in particular. It's much broader than that. The German sociologist Max Weber wrote a classic book at the beginning of the century on the Protestant ethic and the spirit of capitalism. It's about how what have become the dominant religious and economic systems, particularly in northern and western Europe and the U.S., are all built on quite individualistic egos. The prominence of individualistic views in psychology is another example of that, but it's really quite a pervasive phenomenon that cuts across religion, politics, economics — all aspects of human life. I think that the globalization of the world is now making people much more aware of the fact that other people think about and do things rather differently, down to the level where some of the things we once thought were fundamental, inherent properties of human beings turn out to be social and cultural variables.

"There is some quite interesting and powerful stuff coming out of comparative social psychology. For example, it suggests that in a whole range of ways, people in the U.S. and in western European countries are much more individualistic in the way we process information and in the way that we think about relationships. For example, in Asian societies, things are almost immediately considered not just from the perspective of the individual but also from the perspective of the group."

W. Brugh Joy, M.D., is the author of *Joy's Way* and *Avalanche*. He lectures and leads workshops with people who are interested in personal growth, including the value of suffering as a doorway to transformation.

"There is no question, to me, of the sublime value of suffering. The more deeply one has experienced the mystery of suffering, the more deeply one truly understands its transformational power. I believe it transforms the infantile power-drive, which has a sense of unlimitedness, immediacy, self-centeredness, into the mystery of compassion, a sense of 'us,' rather than a sense of 'me versus another.' There is also the mystery of sacrifice, which is a form of suffering in which one gives up one's personal, willful way to something that can only be called transcendent. The experience of this is that the transcendent showers the individual with resources — which may be a healing, or it may be illumination, or it may be compassion. But something that transcends the ordinary comes out of such sacrifices and suffering, which are interwoven."

"In this context, when you sacrifice, are you really sacrificing your sense of being separate and alone?"

"Yes, as long as this addresses the issue of the ego, and particularly the infantile ego, which is immensely self-centered. I see it in simple things, just asking people to consider silence and fasting in the conferences I do. Silence and fasting are a form of sacrifice, and I watch people struggle with it tremendously. You would think that staying silent and surrendering food for two days while still taking in plenty of liquids wouldn't be too hard. And yet many people find it just amazingly difficult. That infantile, instinctual force that gets self-centered — and the idea of going through suffering, the sensation of suffering, of loss, and often anxiety — all these sorts of things around that sacrifice, of not responding to one's immediate gratifications, are difficult. From that initial encounter with sacrifice, if they can reach it, can come some of the most amazing transformations that I've ever encountered with people."

I asked him to describe what he sees when that happens.

"People come into the sense of the realization that there is something greater than themselves, because, suddenly, they are infused with a state of consciousness they know is not their ordinary, egoistic awareness. Rather, it's as if they receive a grace or a blessing. It can only be called somewhat of an epiphany which often occurs when one really approaches the experience with integrity and a sense of reverence. But what the ego experiences is tremendous discomfort, anxiety, and a form of suffering it wants to immediately gratify with something else, so people may abort the process before they get the epiphany. Most of the great religions understand something about the mystery of sacrifice, in terms of the mystery between the ego and the divine essence.

"My experience is that one awakens into degrees of it. One begins to see the larger mystery play of life, that the whole thing is sacred. One sees more of the spiritual dimension of one's profession, more of the sacred dimension, than just the overt, outer, conceptual realization. This awakens them. So, it's like the difference between somebody who is skilled at acting versus somebody who really knows the art, who has come into contact with its deeper forces. You see individuals who are very gifted in their field, as if something is moving them and touching them, and they describe it as something *beyond* themselves, as opposed to technique."

I asked him to describe how relationships are a spiritual path.

"A relationship can be a path of healing, of transformation, but only if you know how to go through the difficulties of relationship as a spiritual path. But rarely is that true, because relationships are usually based more on things that are satisfying the ego, and people haven't differentiated out these deeper experiences and resources. I think what differentiates it is that those individuals are connected to something of a transcendent nature *in* relationship, and that the relationship itself may be the transcendent vehicle. But I find this a very rare development. The more infantile forces are so satisfied in a nourishing relationship, that there may be no stimulation to develop the relationship to the transcendent *in* the relationship. I also know the sublimity of the divine through pathos. So, I want to make sure that there isn't a preference for just joy, but that there is something deeper, where joy and pathos are somehow two sides of the same thing. Therefore, in the relationship, no matter what range it's going to present, the intent is to come to either liberation or a larger sense of being. Somehow, it involves a large range of feeling and emotional responses. Underneath it lies an appreciation or understanding of something that allows one to experience the difficulty *and* to experience the joy in its fullness. That, to me, is what differentiates an infantile relationship, which is only looking for pleasure, from one that is transformative."

"I find it interesting that you started out writing about joy and are now coming to pathos, to realizing that both are necessary."

"This is why I use the phrase 'crisis awakens,' because it's usually through some sort of shock that the psyche begins to realize how superficial their life has been and begins to seek out something more meaningful. Or, it may happen during a serious illness that suddenly they recognize their life may be taken away, and then they become very interested in life again."

James J. Lynch, Ph.D., is the author of *The Broken Heart* and *The Language of the Heart*. He is Professor of Psychiatry at the University of Maryland Medical School and a pioneer in studying the relationship of loneliness to high blood pressure and heart disease.

"In *The Broken Heart*, I described how loneliness is one of the leading causes of death in this country and certainly a major factor in heart disease. It's interesting how words like *loneliness* and *love* were made to disappear from science and medicine, and in their place came phrases like 'mental stress' and 'social support.' There is something about those words that's threatening — *love* is certainly a word that is taboo in science. Charles Darwin, in his book *The Expression of Emotions in Man and Animals: The Study of Fear, Pain, Hunger, Rage, and Love*, said, of all of the emotions, the most powerful is love, but from a scientific perspective, it's the most difficult to study."

I asked him why he thinks this is so.

"I think we have to look at two things, in terms of why this isn't taken seriously by science. The first is that everything within Western medicine's current understanding is framed by the Cartesian model. The entire thrust of modern medicine is mechanisms, the body as a machine. Modern physiology is based on cellular physiology, the belief that cellular regulations are the same in man and animals. And then there is the confusion that Descartes caused by extracting feelings from the body. He created the term emotions, which he considered to be the same in man and in animals — merely chemical perturbations. The only difference was that man had a soul and could decode emotions, so emotions became a property of the soul, not the body. This set the stage for modern medicine.

"The interesting thing is that when I wrote *The Broken Heart*, it was clear that loneliness was a killer. But how do we get from loneliness to high blood pressure or coronary heart disease? We now know at least one of the mechanisms: It was in the discovery of the remarkable blood pressure shifts that happen when we talk. I noticed that every time babies cried, their blood pressure doubled. For a while, I had thought the increase was just a reaction to stress. The longer the babies cried, the higher the blood pressure went. Then it hit me like a lightning bolt one day that the rise in blood pressure was not a response — it was *part* of the communication! Then I realized — that's exactly what the adult patients are doing, but their cries are inward. And I began to understand that listening to people lowers their blood pressure because we hear their cries. I suddenly realized that the way we were looking at the body was limited, that there was a whole other 'body in dialogue' that we had totally overlooked, because we had believed language was separate from the body, as we'd learned from the Cartesian philosophy.

"If you think of the typical patient in modern medicine, they go to a cardiologist, and if there's any chest pain, the cardiologist identifies it, puts them on a treadmill stress test. They go to a hospital where their arteries are bypassed, and, magically, the pain is gone. It seems absolutely clear that it's a matter of plumbing, and the heart is a pump. Now, I ask, who do they think is the *person* occupying all these parts? Then the patient comes to rehabilitation, and what happens? First, they put this *machine* — the patient — on the treadmill, and they get it back in shape. The whole metaphor is mechanical. Then every patient comes to see me, and I hook them up with a blood pressure machine, and minute by minute, we record their pressure.

"We know that blood pressure goes up when you talk. We know it drops when you listen — when you *really* listen. If you think about what you're going to say next while you're listening, it doesn't go back down. And we also know that the higher your baseline pressure is, the more it goes up when you talk. So, if you have already have hypertension, your pressure goes way up when you talk."

I asked, "The blood pressure goes up because the person is overvigilant, afraid that he's not going to be heard, is possibly going to be rejected, or made fun of, or shamed, whereas when they listen they feel connected to the other person?"

"Right. We also found that deaf people, when they sign, do the same thing. So, we know it's not just the talking. It's really the communicating.

"I begin talking with these patients, and I have a monitor going so they can watch the blood pressure changes, minute to minute. But they don't feel any of the changes that are clearly indicated on the monitor. These people know that their pressure goes up when they exercise, and they quickly see that it can go much higher when they talk to me — in spite of any medication they may be on. I suspect that these sudden pressure surges can contribute to the development of coronary atherosclerosis, although that remains to be proven. I have thousands of examples in heart patients.

"So the patients talk while they watch the Dynamap blood pressure machine, and they see their pressure go way up, but they don't feel it. They look at their blood pressure numbers on the machine and ask, 'What's that?' And I say, 'That's you.' And they ask, 'But my blood pressure is 120 over 60 — how can it be 190 over 110?' I say, 'But it's *you.*' I give every patient the same metaphor: 'Suppose you were looking in the mirror and saw your body suddenly expand by fifty percent, and then deflate by fifty percent. Would you be shocked as to who that was in the mirror?' The vascular changes that get fed back during our dialogue are an assault on who they think they are.

"Everyone talks about heart disease being linked to negative emotions, such as anger, depression, and so on. But I view all these internal vascular changes as really hidden forms of communication, like blushing. Blushing is really a hidden form of caring. I blush because I'm afraid I'm going to be rejected, but I care about the other person, and I don't want them to reject me. So, *the vascular changes are the language of the heart* — only they are hidden. Even to a person who cares deeply, this hidden communication can look calm on the surface. It's like a child crying. The greatest risk a baby takes is crying at night, because if there is no mother to respond, then you're dead. Real communication is a life-and-death matter, and so we don't engage in real dialogue very often, because we might be rejected. And when a person tries to talk about something meaningful, the body can explode in terror, because they're terrified that their cry, again, is going to go unheard. What's so interesting is that the greater these changes, the less likely the person is able to feel them."

"Because they are split off from their own feelings?"

"Yes. And they can't detect their own bodies. It's a big, tragic dance. The baby's cry is unheard. And so, the baby, rather than cry out loud, cries inside. Because we do tell people to hide their suffering, their vulnerability and loneliness, and so they also hide their beauty."

I added that when you wall off your capacity to feel pain, you also diminish your capacity to feel pleasure.

"You not only do that, but you wall off your capacity to feel another's pain. Why couldn't the German Nazi doctors hear the cries of those people in the concentration camps? Their narcissism occurred at the cultural level, not just on the individual level. The Master Race, the Beautiful People — these are all narcissistic concepts. My interest in the heart is secondary to more important issues. However we define the individual body is also how we define the body politic of our nation. This is becoming a completely detached, rational, narcissistic society. And by narcissistic, I mean people who are no longer living in their bodies. They can't feel feelings. They are detached from their bodies, and they're living an image. They are living *noplace*. Are you familiar with the concept of narcissism?"

"Yes, I have worked on these issues in my life for a long time."

"Me, too! I was a narcissist for decades without even realizing the problem and never knew it. In fact, I was a full professor at thirty-five. I was absolutely going to fly through life and save the Western world. I never knew that my own writing on loneliness in *The Broken Heart* and *The Language of the Heart* was all autobiographical. I was in search of myself.

"Narcissism, in fact, means *no self*, no *real* self. You live an image which keeps you away from your own body, your own heart. You may appear self-centered, but there is no real self, so therefore you are the world, and there's no boundary. Many people with premature heart disease have significant degrees of narcissism in them. They can't feel their feelings, and so for them love is an ideal, not real. Actually, narcissists are nice people, very sensitive — just very lonely. The problem is, our mothers who taught us to talk struggle with those same issues and suffered in a similar way. They couldn't really see us, so they taught us affective language which couldn't reach us, and so we learned that real talk is problematic. Narcissism is the inability to live in your own body, so you live an image. The journey back home is to come back into your body, into reality, into real feelings. Into your heart."

Gail Gross, Ph.D., holds a doctorate in education with a focus on child psychology. She is a direct descendant of Isaac Luria, considered the father of Kabbalah, an esoteric branch of Judaism. She is the founder of the nation's first residential school for homeless children, located in Houston.

I asked her to describe why loneliness, isolation, anger, and depression predispose to illness and premature death as seen from a Kabbalistic perspective. She discusses these issues in terms of light and dark, familiar themes in many religions and other spiritual paths.

"There's a lesson in the Kabbalah about the oneness of all of us, the connectedness — it's like a connective tissue. We are all connected by a membrane of light. In fact, that is an American Indian concept, too, the idea of the wedding basket: You have a connectedness between mates, that there are membranes of light that tie you to the other. When you are in a healthy relationship, the Kabbalists believe that the light is not obstructed. The Kabbalah lessons are really about simplifying, and even the simplifying is, in itself, a distraction that brings you back to where you already are, to what is already there.

"So, to apply that to a person who is ill, you would say that their clear stream of light is obstructed by blocks or constriction. This is because it takes a lot of energy to hold down secrets, anger, fear, hatred, rejection, grief, to repress what is there. When you remove the constriction, when you are in your heart and you get past the repression, then you are free. Everything is free-flowing. You are light, your immunities go up, you are healthy, because you are in the stream again."

"You're saying that it is like opening a window shade and letting the sunlight in?"

"Yes — the light is always shining, but we are separated from it. In fact, we aren't really separated from anybody, except by our personality or our ego, or what I would call a narcissistic personality. But the acting in separation takes a lot of energy. The use of energy in that way, in a restrictive way, is what makes people unhealthy."

I wondered why acting in separation takes a lot of energy, and why that, in turn, may lead to illness.

"The body itself is not a solid; it just appears to be. It's actually vibrating energy. It vibrates at a certain frequency that makes it appear dense. But, the more you open your heart, the more spiritual you become, the more connected to the light, then the higher the frequency of your resonance. The higher the resonance of the energy, the lighter the body, the healthier the body, because the body is just a construction that houses the soul.

"Take a personality, like a businessman who is very closed and tight, and therefore ill. What is he really doing? Psychologically, he wants to be in control, because he wants things his way. He realizes that if he gives up control, he can't have it all his way. He might be willing to give up a little control and then have it mostly his way and a little bit somebody else's way. But he fears that if he gives up too much control, then somebody will take away everything. So he restricts. He is resonating at a denser, lower level, because he is restricting himself. So instead of being a vessel to take in light, he is constricted, in a sense, closed down, separated from the light. In being separated from the light, you could say he is separated from other people, but really it is from God, from the God within him. So although his conscious mind thinks his life is great, the vessel that was created to hold the light is falling apart, because it can't operate in a healthy way, all clogged and blocked up. He's got to use up his energy to hold down all of the secrets, so he can be the boss, be in control, the big shot. But the irony is, he's killing the very vessel that can give him health and happiness. Life at that level of denseness — except for the momentary highs, which keep the businessmen running for those feelings of 'I'm alive' — is pretty lonely, sad, and difficult, filled with sickness, suffering, and pills. Your friends die, you get old, you lose your potency, your hair falls out, your teeth fall out. They don't want to become that.

"But that's not who they are. The body is just a vessel whose purpose is to house the light, the soul. The soul has to express itself. It has to take a leap of faith, overcoming the fear of moving into something totally unknown.

"Whether you have your total body remade, or build another mansion, or buy another whatever, happiness is not in any of that. It's really all about the light, the idea of imprinting God, like a little duck when it's first born. Whatever shows up in its vision right away is what it imprints on. We were given the imprint on our soul of God. There is God in all of us. The philosophers in the time of Aristotle believed that you only remember what you already knew. It's all there in the DNA of who we are, the DNA of our souls. But we are so busy with life and living and career and mates and children and fighting and importance, and all the things this denser world demands of us. And the criteria that we hold up for success in this life uses us all up.

"Jung would say that all of the defenses — the protective layers — that we have developed to walk through life in a way that makes us feel safe, are constrictions, repressions. They are not the true self, not the individuated self. They are the defended self. We learn that early in our development. There is a disowned part of us — what Jung termed 'the shadow.' But only when you integrate the shadow and embrace it as part of the entire aspect of what it means to be human, only then can you come into fulfillment and individuation. It seems like a paradox, but you first need to feel individuated in order to feel whole, to recognize that you are part of everybody, and that everybody is a part of you. But when you are young, you defend yourself to be safe, and you learn very quickly that you have to cover up the part of you that seems to not be working, like screaming and yelling, and getting mad, and being jealous, or losing your temper. You ultimately repress it or disown it, but like a shadow, it's still there. It's the very repression of that behavior — holding it down — that can make you sick.

"To survive, the shadow must be integrated, because anything that is repressed causes destruction, a breakdown. The repression or the holding down of the shadow may lead to illness. But, it is the real self, the undefended self that is always fine, happy, light."

I added that when you can be with someone whom you can trust and show your shadow and still feel loved, it's like shining a light in the darkness; the ability of the shadow to influence us diminishes and we have less need to project our shadow onto other people.

"Jung talks about a soldier who is torturing a victim. We are in horror at the idea of this, but when we break through, psychologically and spiritually, we realize that inside each of us there is also a torturer. When we realize this, by a dream or an experience, then we feel peaceful and light, because it's integrated. This is a merging of dream and awake time; we are aware of the shadow while awake, not just when dreaming. We think to ourselves, 'Ah-ha! Yes. That also is me. Therefore, I don't have to act it out, I don't have to repress it.'"

I said, "That is the essence of compassion."

"Yes, it takes away the separation. Then you think, 'Oh, that's how we all are.' No more separation. We ultimately start isolating ourselves, because we fear people are going to take something away from us. This has to do with the shadow, because the shadow was taken from us when we were children by our parents. They said that not only won't we be lovable, but we will be punished if we have it. They said, 'It's inappropriate to wet your pants or play with yourself or fight, hit your brother, break something,' whatever. The child hears, 'I'm not going to love you,' and 'I am going to punish you.' So, we now have two things happening that we do to ourselves. We don't integrate the shadow, but we do internalize our parents. When we become adults, we hear the voice of mother and father merged. We decide we are not lovable, and then we punish ourselves, because the shadow is there. The punishing keeps us in isolation and it breaks down the body. For example, what is depression but anger turned inward? We punish ourselves because our shadow is acting it out. But when you accept the shadow as an adult, you don't have to act it out.

"In ancient Hebrew, they say that you should fear God, but the word *fear* really means *awe*, that you should be in awe of God, because in the end, you should do all these things, not because you are afraid, not because you want things for yourself, but simply because you are pleasing God, as well as yourself. You are receiving for the sake of sharing and therefore imitating God — being like God. Rather than *my* will be done, it becomes '*Thy* will be done.' We lose our separateness and loneliness and realize God."

I replied, "It seems that whatever discipline or religion you are part of, if you take it far enough, you may end up in a similar place — only with a different language to try to make sense out of it.

"Because you are really there already."

Larry Dossey, M.D., is a pioneering physician who is the editor of the journal *Alter-*

native Therapies in Health and Medicine. He is the author of several books, including *Healing Words.*

I asked Dr. Dossey why he thinks love and intimacy are such powerful determinants of health.

"I've asked myself this question many times, and as far as I can tell, there are two ways of approaching this. One does not raise any eyebrows and doesn't create much intellectual indigestion. This is the mechanistic way of understanding how these things operate. For instance, the value of religion and religious practice is attributed to a better diet, avoidance of tobacco and alcohol, stress management, increased social contact at church, and so on. I don't know many people who would object to that type of analysis any more, in this emerging age of mind-body medicine. I think that approach to trying to understand how these things come about can take us only so far."

Dr. Dossey believes that the question of why love and intimacy play such an important role in health and healing is not fully answerable within the current models of science. "Personally, I think that we just are going to have to bite the bullet and get out of this mechanistic box if we're going to understand how these things operate. I see

442

no way around invoking new concepts of consciousness to explain these effects.

"Now, what I am about to say is outrageous, but I've thought about this an awfully long time. I think that there are interpersonal, nonlocal, consciousness-mediated events through which one individual can influence another individual's health. I think there is compelling evidence that such an extended model of consciousness and interpersonal influence is going to be necessary.

"People are floundering around, trying to find a rather nonthreatening vocabulary with which to talk about this. One of the terms that is floating to the top is *distant intentionality,* which is one of Dr. Marilyn Schlitz's favorite terms. If one is willing to put preconceptions aside and simply look at the data and the quality of experiments, I think one sees a sobering picture developing. It may be possible for me to influence the status of your health through loving, compassionate mental intentions, thoughts, and wishes (such as prayer) at a distance, even when you are unaware I am doing that. This has been shown in admirable experiments, involving not just human beings, where these events are typically explained away in terms of placebo responses, but also in lower organisms.

"These studies have been done with fanatical precision looking at growth rates of bacteria, fungi, plants, germination rates of seeds, healing of wounds in rats and mice, and so on. They show clearly, in my judgment, that the empathic, loving thoughts of one individual can affect a distant biological system. There is no way that these events can be explained in terms of suggestion, expectations, placebo responses, and so forth, since they have been replicated not just in humans, but in lower organisms as well.

"There is a section in my book *Healing Words* that lists 130 of those studies. It's all too easy for cynics and skeptics to draw a bead on these. One can always find poorly done studies in a field this sprawling. There are also fanatically precise studies in this field. If one looks at the best data, I think you can paint a compelling picture for nonlocal expressions of consciousness and intention.

"I get hundreds of letters from people describing remarkable cures from serious illnesses. Usually these cases involve the use of *both* prayer and orthodox medical procedures. It is truly rare that someone writes me about using *only* prayer. These letters fascinate me, because they show that when Americans get sick they are extremely pragmatic. They like to cover all their bases when they get sick. They choose prayer *and* penicillin, which I think is a very healthy response to the issues we've been discussing.

"I think we are on the verge of a fabulous new understanding of how we interact with each other, and what we cavalierly call 'social support' these days will be understood as something much more complex and majestic in the future."

I replied that even with the idea of non-local influence, the question remains of what's really happening. "Whether it's you and I talking across the phone or in person, or I'm praying for you. Why is that healing?"

"The main issue, theoretically, at this stage, is to develop a model that permits the phenomenon. I'll tell you what David Chalmers says. He wrote an article in *Scientific American*, December 1995, called "The Puzzle of Conscious Experience." The bottom line of his paper is that it is time for us to simply bite the bullet and declare that consciousness is fundamental in the universe, on a par with matter and energy. Now, I agree that it's tempting to ask how consciousness works — as you have asked, 'How does this happen?' But there is a certain level in scientific progress where one simply swallows a great idea and becomes so comfortable with it that asking questions about how it happened seems to feel less important."

"An analogy can be made with the idea of universal gravity, which, when Newton introduced it in the 1600s, was condemned as utterly mystical. No one could explain why it happened, why bodies would behave that way. And *since* then, no one has explained it."

In other words, I said, we can *describe* gravity even though we do not *understand* it. Even when we do not understand all of the mechanisms by which gravity — or love and intimacy — have such a powerful effect on us, we can still describe the observed phenomena.

"Exactly. But you would be thought odd today if you questioned universal gravity. So, there's a sense in which we simply get used to new concepts; eventually they come to seem self-obvious. Gravity is like that, and I suspect that the mechanism of consciousness will be like that, too. I loved Chalmers's proposal that consciousness is a fundamental factor in the universe like matter and energy. This is not an Oriental mystic talking, yet you cannot separate the gist of his suggestion from a mystical model.

"There are a lot of theoretical scientists of Nobel caliber around the world thinking about this question you are raising — how does this happen? How are we to think about this? Is this permissible? Brian Josephson, a Nobel Prize–winning physicist, has suggested in an article in *Foundations of Physics*, one of the most prestigious physics journals, that these interpersonal, nonlocal influences, such as prayer, telepathy, precognition, and so on, will be explainable through advances in our understanding of the concept of nonlocality in quantum mechanics. Another recent proposal has come from the systems theorist Ervin Laszlo, who wrote a book called *The Interconnected Universe.* His proposal is that a development in the field of physics called the *quantum vacuum,* explains these distant intentional events."

I wondered if we can we find common ground between the mystical and the scientific.

"Yes. I must say that I felt at home with these general conclusions from a mystical, Eastern point of view a long time before I ever knew they could be supported through empirical data. But I don't think we can settle for a mystical insight. In our culture, whether any of us likes it or not, the power of science is too pervasive. At some point, if possible, we will have to marry our mystical intuitions about the nature of consciousness with scientific empiricism. I think that if that can be done — and I don't think, like many scientists, we're that far away from it. I hesitate to say that publicly, because when scientists hear the word *mysticism,* they have all sorts of inappropriate responses to it.

"We will have to marry our mystical intuitions about the nature of consciousness with scientific empiricism. The pendulum in our culture has swung so far to the side of mechanism and determinism and physicalism that one could almost predict an emerging hunger — in medicine, and in our culture at large — for something more nourishing, something more spiritual. And I think we are seeing the evidence that the pendulum is swinging toward the other side. What we need to avoid, however, are these wild oscillations. Your work and mine, and many other people's work, can be seen as an attempt to dampen these oscillations to some sensible middle ground, where we honor reason and intellect as well as intuition and spirituality. That is where I hope we wind up."

We end where we started, with love and survival. Let's give the epilogue to the Sufi poet Rumi, who lived in the thirteenth century when he wrote:

There is a community of the spirit.
Join it, and feel the delight
of walking in the noisy street,
and *being* the noise. . . .
Why do you stay in prison
when the door is so wide open?
Move outside the tangle of fear-thinking.
Live in silence.
Flow down and down in always
widening rings of being.

Acknowledgments

It is one of life's ironies that writing a book on the healing power of love and intimacy has caused me to spend so much time alone in front of a computer. I am thankful for all the people who excused my absence during the time I was writing.

The longer I do this work, the more aware I become of a sublime paradox: I need to act as though everything I do is dependent on my actions while recognizing at the same time that it is all beyond my control. When I stop for a moment to notice this and to reflect on how much support I have received from so many different people and places, both known and unknown, I am overwhelmed with gratitude. So much grace surrounds us all the time if we just pay attention to it.

I hardly know where to begin. Diane Reverand and her colleagues at HarperCollins Publishers showed great confidence in me by enabling me to do this book and enormous patience in waiting for my personal life to catch up with my clinical experience so that I could complete the book. Diane is an editor's editor, and I feel very fortunate to have been able to work with her. I am also very appreciative of others at HarperCollins who made this book possible, including Anthea Disney, David Steinberger, Jack McKeown, Rick Pracher, Doreen Louie, Steven Sorrentino, Stephanie Lehrer, David Flora, Marilyn Allen, Carl Raymond, Craig Herman, Claire Griffin, Frank Fochetta, Richard Rhorer, Daniel Blackman, Anne Gaudinier, and others. My appreciation and respect for Esther Newberg and for Michael Rudell and his associates continues to grow over time. Additional valued counsel was provided by Joel Goldman and Bob Lieber. Donna Gould and Arielle Ford disseminate information better than anyone, and Stacey Kennington at Omega Travel is a travel wizard. I am very grateful to Vivian Glyck for coordinating all of the related activities. Thanks to Karen Gnat and Rick Hassen at Conscious Wave, Julie Kahn and Vicki Schlessinger at Fleishman-Hillard, to Duke Tufty and Patty Porter at the Cornerstone Foundation, and to Harry Rhoads, Jr., Karin March, and Michael Menchel at the Washington Speakers Bureau.

The extraordinary cover art is by Laurel Burch, who also transforms her life into a work of art.

Several people read the manuscript in various stages and made helpful comments. These include Alan Arkin, Dr. Jim Billings, Judy Toran Cousin, Dr. Bob Cunnion, Laura Dern, Drs. Rachelle and Terry Doody, Dr. William Fair, Woody Fraser, Gail Gross, Peter Guber, Mary Hager, Bob Lieber, Dr. Lee Lipsenthal, Terri Merritt, Phillip Moffitt, Dr. Jeremy Nobel, Dr. Edwin and Natalie Ornish, Dr. Steven and Marty Ornish, Laurel Ornish, Dr. Rachel Remen, Michael Rudell, David Salzman, Janet Schreiber, Linda Stone, Dr. Andrew Weil, Will Weinstein, and others.

For the past fourteen years, my colleagues and I at the nonprofit Preventive Medicine Research Institute (PMRI) have conducted a series of clinical research studies and demonstration projects, many of which I described earlier in this book. PMRI has been an opportunity for me to create and work with a community of people who have the rare qualities of being caring and compassionate as well as extremely competent and passionately committed to service.

Dr. Jim Billings is a visionary who has been in charge of the day-to-day operations at PMRI. More than that, he is like the older brother I never had; in his words, we are joined at the hip. Along the same lines, Dr. Lee Lipsenthal refers to himself as a younger brother, and I appreciate his passion for music as well as his love of medicine.

Other colleagues now at PMRI include Heather Amador, Bob Avenson, Marcia Billings, Dr. Richard J. Brand, Courtney Breed, Judy Toran Cousin, Nischala Devi, Melanie Elliott, Jordan Fein, Matthew Fritts, Jean-Marc Fullsack, Amy Gage, Michael Hall, Jeanmaire Hryshko, Dennis Malone, Dr. Ruth Marlin, Patty McCormac, Myrna Melling, Terri Merritt, Laura Nugent, Jean Opipari, Glenn Perelson, Dr. Elaine Pettengill, Ari Pugliese, Caren Raisin, Ana Regalia, Dr. Larry Scherwitz, Janet Schreiber, Lynne Twist, and Bryce Williams. I am especially indebted to Marjorie McClain, who has organized my at times chaotic life for many years. Also, I remain thankful for everyone else who has worked at PMRI in the past.

I am very grateful for the PMRI board members, including Henry Groppe, Jenard Gross, Gerald Hines, Steve Jobs, and Fenton Talbott. I deeply appreciate the members of the PMRI Scientific Advisory Board, including Dr. Christine Cassel, Dr. William Fair, Dr. David Kessler, Dr. C. Everett Koop, Dr. Alexander Leaf (who continues to be an inspiring mentor for me), and Dr. William C. Roberts.

In a real sense, this book draws on all of the clinical and research experience I gained from all of the studies that my colleagues and I have conducted. These studies would not have been possible without the generous support provided by a number of individuals, foundations, and organizations during the past twenty years.

Major support was provided by: The Bucksbaum Family (Martin, Melva, Mary, Matthew, and Kay), Steve and Laurene Jobs, Larry Ellison, Linda Wachner, David Koch, Stewart and Lynda Resnick, the National Heart, Lung, and Blood Institute of the National Institutes of Health (including Drs. Claude Lenfant, Lawrence Friedman, Jeffrey Cutler, Peter Kaufmann, and Stephen Weiss), the Department of Health Services of the State of California, Norman and Lyn Lear, Robert Lehman/The Fetzer Institute, Ken and Linda Lay/The Enron Foundation, the Henry J. Kaiser Family Foundation, Jack Weekly/Mutual of Omaha, Houston Endowment Inc., Gerald and Barbara Hines, Michael Milken/CapCURE, Charles Stine/The Montgomery Street Foundation, Al and Celia Weatherhead, Will Weinstein/Jewish Community Foundation, Brian and Diana Taussig, Mary Smart/The Smart Foundation, Marvin and Marie Bomer, Arthur Andersen & Co., Charles Halperin/The Nathan Cummings Foundation, Frank Lorenzo/ Continental Airlines, Jay and Cindy Pritzker/ The Pritzker Family, Richard Goldman/The Goldman Fund, Paul Glenn/The Glenn Foundation, Don and Doris Fisher/The Gap Foundation, The Ray C. Fish Foundation, Siva Sankaran, Howard and Mary Lester/ Lester Family Foundation, M. B. Seretean Foundation, Norman and Gerry Sue Arnold/ Arnold Foundation, ConAgra Inc., Avram Miller, The First Boston Corporation, Ben Love/Texas Commerce Bank, The Emde Company, The Phyllis and Stuart Moldaw Philanthropic Fund, Drexel Burnham Lambert, Transco Energy Co., Lee Stein, Alan Patricof/New York Community Trust, Corrine and David R. Gould, Dick and Kathy Dawson, Paul Wenner, Dede and Al Wilsey, Benny and Adele Alagem, Brooke and Shawn Byers, Mickey and Peggy Drexler, Henry and Carol Groppe, Jenard and Gail Gross.

Additional supporters include: Sandy Climan, Victoria Greenleaf, Barbara and Gerson Bakar, Robert Graham, American Express, First Church of Danvers, Odyssey Partners, Quaker Oats, Melvin Simon, Susan Franzheim/The Franzheim Synergy Trust, Herberger's, General Growth Companies, Goldman Sachs, Citibank Delaware, Wornick Family Foundation, David and Mary Robinson, Pat Burns, Ken Hubbard and Tori Dauphiont, Kandi Amelon, The Ziegler Corporation, William Davis, Lita and Morton Heller Foundation, William and Flora Hewlett Foundation, McNulty Foundation, Robert Finnell and Marianne Pallotti, Harold Grinspoon, James Langdon, Jeffrey Rhodes, Margoes Foundation, George Harris, Simon and Paula Young, Robert and Karen Lovejoy, Johnson and Johnson, Dr. Edwin and Natalie Ornish, Hans Mautner/Corporate Property Investors, Edward Ehlers, Carl Stevens, Alan and Carol Feren, John and Carol McCaughan, Ira Ingerman, Penny Ferrara, Alfred Heller, Paul Thionville, Peter and Lisa Douglas/ Douglas Foundation, Louise Gartner/Jewish Federation of Greater Dallas, Frank Liddle/ Greater Houston Community Foundation, E. Geraldine Fisher, Hugh R. Goodrich, Edward O. Gaylord, Fayez Sarofim & Co., Eileen Rockefeller Growald/the Institute for the Advancement of Health, Dr. Lucy Rockefeller Waletzky, Eleanor and John Winthrop, Biopsychosocial Research Fund of the Medical Illness Counseling Center, United Energy Resources, The Duncan Foundation (John Duncan), Mesa Petroleum, Brown & Root, Inc., U.S. Venture Partners, The Sackman Foundation, Dr. Jack Bagshaw/Physis Health Center, Leo Fields Family Philanthropic Fund, Bill and Uta Bone, Dr. and Mrs. James Langdon, William and Lucero Meyer, T. B. Hudson, the Bob Hope International Heart Research Institute, Arnold and Carol Ablon, Dr. Pat McKenna, Werner and Eva Hebenstreit, Mel and Lenore Lefer, Amos and Dorian Krausz, Robert McAleese, Thomas Russell Potts, Victor and Lydia Karpenko, Simon and Paula Young, Doug Hawley, Van Gordon Sauter, PPG Industries, Burton Kaufman, James and Margaret Keith, Howard B. Wolf & Co., Joseph Frelinghuysen, Edward F. Kunin, David Harrison, Dr. Kit Peterson, Joseph Forgione, and the Institute of Noetic Sciences. Please forgive me and let me know if I left anyone out who supported our work and I will include their name in the next edition.

Each year since 1984, Arthur Anderson & Co. has provided a complete financial audit of the Preventive Medicine Research Institute on a pro bono basis, for which we remain deeply grateful.

I am very grateful to each person that I interviewed for chapter 6 of this book: Dr. Lisa Berkman, Dr. Jim Billings, Dr. Joan

Borysenko, Dr. Larry Dossey, Dr. Dan Goleman, Dr. John Gray, Gail Gross, T. George Harris, Dr. James House, Dr. Brugh Joy, Dr. Jon Kabat-Zinn, Rob Lehman, Stephen and Ondrea Levine, Dr. James Lynch, Dr. Jacqueline McCandless, Dr. Richard Moss, Carol Naber, Dr. Kristina Orth-Gomér, Dr. Candace Pert, Dr. Rachel Remen, Sri Swami Satchidananda, Dr. Gary Schwartz, Dr. S. Leonard Syme, Dr. Robert A. F. Thurman, Dr. Redford Williams, and Dr. Harvey Zarren. I appreciate Nancy Marriott for helping to edit these transcripts. Also, many thanks to Vivekan Flint for help in obtaining journal articles.

I admire and appreciate Dr. Haile T. Debas (Chancellor and Dean at the School of Medicine, University of California, San Francisco), and Lee Goldman, M.D. (Chairman, Department of Medicine and Associate Dean for Clinical Affairs) for their vision and leadership in establishing the Center for Integrative Medicine at UCSF. I am thankful for the opportunity to work with Dr. Ellen Hughes, Dr. Laura Esserman, Dr. Rachel Remen, Dr. Andy Avins, Dr. Nancy Adler, Joyce McKinney, Jan Rogerson, Mary Tagliaferri, Malka Gorman, and others who are making this vision a reality,

459

including Dr. William Grossman, Martha Hooven, Cindy Lima, Bruce Schroffel, Dr. Bruce Wintroub, Dr. William Margaretten, and others. Part of the Center for Integrative Medicine includes the UCSF/California Pacific Medical Center Program for Reversing Heart Disease, which would not be possible without the above people plus Dr. Martin Brotman, Dr. Allan Pont, Dr. Bruce Brent, Dr. Anne Thorson, Kevin Worth, and their colleagues.

I am very grateful to the administration and staffs of the other hospitals in our demonstration network. These include everyone at Alegent Medical Center (Immanuel Hospital and Bergin Mercy Hospital) in Omaha, Scripps Clinic and Hospitals in La Jolla, Iowa Heart Center/Mercy Hospital in Des Moines, Richland Memorial Hospital in Columbia, South Carolina, Highmark/Blue Cross Blue Shield in Pittsburgh, Broward General Hospital in Ft. Lauderdale. Other hospitals that have contributed to our demonstration project include Beth Israel Deaconess Medical Center at Harvard Medical School in Boston, Mt. Diablo Hospital in Concord, California, and Beth Israel Medical Center in New York. I remain grateful to Dr. Alexander Leaf and his colleagues at the data coordinating center at the Massachusetts General Hospital, including Dr. David Schoenfeld and Judy Scheer.

Other institutions that have collaborated on our studies during the past twenty years include Baylor College of Medicine, The Methodist Hospital, St. Luke's Hospital, the University of California, Berkeley, and the University of Texas Medical School, Houston.

I appreciate so much the opportunity to collaborate with Dr. Peter Carroll at UCSF, Dr. William Fair at Memorial Sloan-Kettering Cancer Center, and my colleagues at PMRI on a randomized, controlled trial to determine if the progression of prostate cancer may be slowed, stopped, or perhaps even reversed by making comprehensive lifestyle changes.

Perhaps most important, my colleagues and I are extremely grateful to everyone who has participated and who is currently participating in any of our research or demonstration projects. Without these brave and dedicated pioneers, none of our studies and none of my books — including this one — would have been possible. We owe them a tremendous debt of gratitude.

I am very grateful to everyone at the Health Care Financing Administration for conducting a review of our program as a cost-effective alternative to bypass surgery and angioplasty for selected patients and to the many people who supported this process. I hope that this will make comprehensive lifestyle changes available to those who most need and can least afford to make them.

Having seen what a powerful difference changes in diet and lifestyle can make in the lives of so many people, I appreciate everyone at ConAgra, Golden Valley, and related companies who have made possible a new line of foods, ADVANTAGE/10, that make it easier and more convenient for people to eat this way. These include Bruce Rohde, Jack McKeon (thanks also for the nonfat popcorn that helped to fuel this book), Mike Trautschold, Bill Welsh, Bill Norton, Carson Burke, Lynn Phares, and many others.

I am deeply appreciative to Michael Schwarz, Peter Stein, Tony Greco, and Jimmy Scalem for making possible the PBS series based on this book.

I look forward to working together with Mark Pacala and his colleagues at American Whole Health to make our work more widely available.

I appreciate Phil Lader and Linda Le-Sourd Lader for establishing Renaissance Weekend, a wonderful example of the power of community that I describe in this book.

I remain very grateful for the friendship of President Clinton and Hillary Rodham Clinton and for the vision and leadership they provide our country as we approach a new millennium.

I deeply love my parents, Dr. Edwin and Natalie Ornish, and appreciate the many sacrifices they made on my behalf. I am especially grateful for their blessing in allowing me to write about some personal issues in chapter 3 involving them. I appreciate and love my siblings — Laurel, Steven (and his wife Marty), and Kathy (and her husband John). Sri Swami Satchidananda has been an ongoing source of inspiration, friendship, and guidance during the past twenty-five years. As described in chapter 3, I owe my survival to him, for which words of appreciation are inadequate. Dr. Gary Burstein also has made a profound difference in the process of my ongoing development.

Most of all, I want to thank Molly Blackwell, to whom I have dedicated this book — and my life.

I am very grateful for the opportunity to have written this book, which has been very meaningful for me. I hope you have found at least some of it to be useful.

Notes

Chapter 1: Love and Survival

1. Spiegel, D., J. R. Bloom, H. C. Kraemer, and E. Gottheil. "Effect of psychosocial treatment on survival of patients with metastatic breast cancer." *The Lancet*, 1989, ii:888–91.
2. Eisenberg, D. "Unconventional medicine in the United States." *New England Journal of Medicine*, 1993, 328(4):282–83.
3. Ornish D. M., L. W. Scherwitz, R. S. Doody, et al. "Effects of stress management training and dietary changes in treating ischemic heart disease." *Journal of the American Medical Association*, 1983, 249:54–59.
4. Ornish, D. M., S. E. Brown, L. W. Scherwitz, et al. "Can lifestyle changes reverse coronary atherosclerosis? The Lifestyle Heart Trial." *The Lancet*, 1990, 336:129–33. (Reprinted in *Yearbook of Medicine* and *Yearbook of Cardiology* New York: C.V. Mosby, 1991).

5. Gould, K. L., D. Ornish, L. Scherwitz, et al. "Changes in myocardial perfusion abnormalities by positron emission tomography after long-term, intense risk factor modification." *Journal of the American Medical Association*, 1995, 274:894–901.

6. Gould, K. L., D. Ornish, R. Kirkeeide, S. Brown, et al. "Improved stenosis geometry by quantitative coronary arteriography after vigorous risk factor modification." *American Journal of Cardiology*, 1992, 69:845–53.

7. Ornish, D. M., A. M. Gotto, R. R. Miller, et al. "Effects of a vegetarian diet and selected yoga techniques in the treatment of coronary heart disease." *Clinical Research*, 1979, 27:720A.

8. Scherwitz, L., and D. Ornish. "The impact of major lifestyle changes on coronary stenosis, CHD risk factors, and psychological status: results from the San Francisco Lifestyle Heart Trial." *Homeostasis*, 1994, 35:190–204.

9. Ornish, D. "Reversing heart disease through diet, exercise, and stress management." *Journal of the American Dietetic Association*, 1991, 91:162–65.

10. Ornish, D. "Can lifestyle changes reverse coronary atherosclerosis?" *Hospi-*

tal Practice, May 1991.

11. Ornish, D. "Can you prevent — and reverse — coronary artery disease?" *Patient Care*, 1991, 25:25–41.

12. Ornish, D. "Can atherosclerosis regress?" *Cardiovascular Risk Factors*, 1992, 2(4):276–81.

13. Dienstfrey, H. "What makes the heart healthy? A talk with Dean Ornish." *Advances*, 1992, 8(2):25–45.

14. Barnard, N., L. Scherwitz, and D. Ornish. "Adherence and acceptability of a low-fat, vegetarian diet among cardiac patients." *Journal of Cardiopulmonary Rehabilitation*, 1992, 12:423–31.

15. Ornish, D. "Can lifestyle changes reverse coronary heart disease?" *World Review of Nutrition and Dietetics*, 1993, 72:38–48.

16. Ornish, D. "Lessons from the Lifestyle Heart Trial." *Choices in Cardiology*, 1991, 1(5):1–4.

17. Ornish, D. M. "Stress and coronary heart disease: new concepts." In *For Your Health*, ed. R. J. Carlson and B. Newman. New York: C. V. Mosby, 1987.

18. Ornish, D. "Dietary saturated fatty acids and low-density or high-density lipoprotein cholesterol." *New England*

Journal of Medicine, 1990, 322:403.
19. Ornish, D. "What if Americans ate less fat?" *Journal of the American Medical Association*, 1992, 267(3):362.
20. Ornish, D. "Dietary treatment of hyperlipidemia." *Journal of Cardiovascular Risk*, 1994, 1:283–86.
21. Moyers, Bill. "Changing Life Habits: A Conversation with Dean Ornish." In *Healing and the Mind*. New York: Doubleday, 1993.
22. Ornish, D., and S. E. Brown. "Treatment of and screening for hyperlipidemia." *New England Journal of Medicine*, 1993, 329(15):1124–25.
23. Ornish, D. "Can lifestyle changes reverse coronary heart disease?" In *Multiple Risk Factors in Cardiovascular Disease, 2nd Symposium Proceedings*. Tokyo: Churchill Livingstone Japan, 1994, pp. 53–60.
24. Billings, J., L. Scherwitz, R. Sullivan, and D. Ornish. "Group support therapy in the Lifestyle Heart Trial." In S. Scheidt and R. Allan, eds. *Heart and Mind: The Emergence of Cardiac Psychology*. Washington, D.C.: American Psychological Association, 1996, pp. 233–53.
25. Curtin, M. E. *Symposium on Love*. New

York: Behavioral Publications, 1973.

26. Joeg, J. M. "Evaluating coronary heart disease risk: tiles in the mosaic." *Journal of the American Medical Association*, 1997, 277:1387–90.

27. Mumford, D. "Thank God I have cancer." *Journal of the American Medical Association*, 1997, 278:965.

28. Wines, M. "Cabinet memoir discovers humans in masks of power." *New York Times*. March 30, 1997, section 1, p. 1.

Chapter 2: The Scientific Basis for the Healing Power of Intimacy

1. Greenwood, D. C., K. R. Muir, C. J. Packham, et al. "Coronary heart disease: a review of the role of psychosocial stress and social support." *Journal of Public Health Medicine*, 1996, 18:221–31.

2. Russek, L. G., and G. E. Schwartz. "Feelings of parental caring predict health status in midlife: a 35-year follow-up of the Harvard Mastery of Stress Study." *Journal of Behavioral Medicine*, 1997, 20:1–13.

3. Seeman, T. E., and S. L. Syme. "Social networks and coronary artery disease: a comparison of the structure and func-

tion of social relations as predictors of disease." *Psychosomatic Medicine*, 1987, 49(4):341–54.

4. Horsten, M., R. Kirkeeide, B. Svane, K. Schenck-Gustafsson, M. Blom, S. Wamala, and K. Orth-Gomér. Social support and coronary artery disease in women. Personal communication.

5. Medalie, J. H., and U. Goldbourt. "Angina pectoris among 10,000 men. II. Psychosocial and other risk factors as evidenced by a multivariate analysis of a five year incidence study." *American Journal of Medicine*, 1976, 60(6): 910–21.

6. Medalie, J. H., K. C. Stange, S. J. Zyzanski, and U. Goldbourt. "The importance of biopsychosocial factors in the development of duodenal ulcer in a cohort of middle-aged men." *American Journal of Epidemiology*, 1992, 136(10):1280–87.

7. Orth-Gomér, K., and A. L. Undén. "The measurement of social support in population surveys." *Soc. Sci Med.*, 1987, 24:83–94.

8. Orth-Gomér, K., A. Rosengren, and L. Wilhelmsen. "Lack of social support and incidence of coronary heart disease

in middle-aged Swedish men." *Psychosomatic Medicine*, 1993, 55:37–43.

9. Helgeson, V. S., and S. Cohen. "Social support and adjustment to cancer." *Health Psychology*, 1996, 15:135–48.

10. Amick, T. L., and J. K. Ockene. "The role of social support in the modification of risk factors for cardiovascular disease." In Sally A. Shumaker and Susan M. Czajkowski, eds., *Social Support and Cardiovascular Disease*. New York: Plenum Press, 1994.

11. Cohen, S. "Psychosocial models of the role of social support in the etiology of physical disease." *Health Psychology*, 1988, 7:269–97.

12. Cobb, S. Presidential Address — 1976. "Social support as a moderator of life stress." *Psychosomatic Medicine*, 1976, 38(5):300–314.

13. Ornish, D. *Eat More, Weigh Less*. New York: HarperCollins Publishers, 1993.

14. Depner, C. E., and Ingersoll-Dayton. "Supportive relationships in later life." *Psychology and Aging*, 1988, 3:348–57.

15. Cassileth, B. R., E. J. Lusk, D. S. Miller, et al. "Psychosocial correlates of survival in advanced malignant disease." *New England Journal of Medicine*, 1985, 312:1551–55.

16. Rhinegold, H. *The Virtual Community.* New York: HarperCollins Publishers, 1994.

17. Selye, H. *The Stress of Life.* New York: McGraw-Hill, 1976.

18. Holmes, T. H. "Multidiscipline studies of tuberculosis." In P. Sparer, ed., *Personality, Stress, and Tuberculosis.* New York: International Universities Press, 1956.

19. Berkman, L. F. "The role of social relations in health promotion." *Psychosomatic Medicine,* 1995, 57:245–54.

20. Russek, L. G., and G. E. Schwartz. "Perceptions of parental caring predict health status in midlife: a 35-year follow-up of the Harvard Mastery of Stress Study." *Psychosomatic Medicine,* 1997, 59(2):144–49.

21. Funkenstein, D., S. King, and M. Drolette. *Mastery of Stress.* Cambridge, MA: Harvard University Press, 1957.

22. Russek, L. G., and G. E. Schwartz. "Narrative descriptions of parental love and caring predict health status in midlife: a 35-year follow-up of the Harvard Mastery of Stress Study." *Alternative Therapies in Health and Medicine,* 1996, 2:55–62.

23. Thomas, C. B., and K. R. Duszynski.

"Closeness to parents and the family constellation in a prospective study of five disease states: suicide, mental illness, malignant tumor, hypertension, and coronary heart disease." *Johns Hopkins Medical Journal*, 1974, 134: 251.

24. Graves, P. L., C. B. Thomas, and L. A. Mead. "Familial and psychological predictors of cancer." *Cancer Detection & Prevention*, 1991, 15(1):59–64.

25. Lynch, J. J. *The Broken Heart: The Medical Consequences of Loneliness.* New York: Basic Books, 1977.; Baltimore: Bancroft Press, 1998.

26. Shaffer, J. W., K. R. Duszynski, and C. B. Thomas. "Family attitudes in youth as a possible precursor of cancer among physicians: a search for explanatory mechanisms." *Journal of Behavioral Medicine*, 1982, 5(2):143–63.

27. Syme, S. L. Conference on Behavioral Medicine and Cardiovascular Disease: Coronary artery disease: a sociocultural perspective. *Circulation*, Supplement 1, 1987, 76(1): I112-I116. American Heart Association Monograph 6.

28. Durkheim, E. *Suicide.* New York: Free Press, 1951.

29. Kissen, D. M. "The significance of personality in lung cancer in men." *Annals of the New York Academy of Sciences*, 1966, 125(3):820–26.
30. Kissen, D. M., R. I. Brown, and M. Kissen. "A further report on personality and psychosocial factors in lung cancer." *Annals of the New York Academy of Sciences*, 1969, 164(2): 535–45.
31. Russek, L. G., and G. E. Schwartz. "Family love and lifelong health? A challenge for psychology and society." *American Psychologist.* In press.
32. Friedman, S. B., L. A. Glasgow, and R. Ader. "Psychological factors modifying host resistance to experimental infections." *Annals of the New York Academy of Sciences*, 1969, 164: 381–93.
33. Ader, R., and S. B. Friedman. "Some social factors affecting emotionality and resistance to disease in animals. V: Early separation from the mother and response to a transplanted tumor in the rat." *Psychosomatic Medicine*, 1965, 27:119–22.
34. McCauley, J., D. E. Kern, K. Kolodner, et al. "Clinical characteristics of women with a history of childhood

abuse." *Journal of the American Medical Association*, 1997, 277:1362–68.

35. Parker, G. P., E. A. Barrett, and I. B. Hickie. "From nurture to network: examining links between perceptions of parenting received in childhood and social bonds in adulthood." *American Journal of Psychiatry*, 1992, 149: 877–85.

36. Vaillant, G. E. "Natural history of male psychological health. VI: correlates of successful marriage and fatherhood." *American Journal of Psychiatry*, 1978, 135:653–59.

37. Parker, G. P., E. A. Barrett, and I. B. Hickie. "From nurture to network: examining links between perceptions of parenting received in childhood and social bonds in adulthood." *American Journal of Psychiatry*, 1992, 149: 877–85.

38. Egolf, B., J. Lasker, S. Wolf, and L. Potvin. "Featuring health risks and mortality: the Roseto effect: a 50-year comparison of mortality rates." *American Journal of Public Health*, 1992, 82(8):1089–92.

39. Wolf, S. "Predictors of myocardial infarction over a span of 30 years in Roseto, Pennsylvania." *Integrative*

Physiological & Behavioral Science,
1992, 27(3):246–57.
40. Berkman, L. F., and S. L. Syme. "Social networks, host resistance, and mortality: a nine-year follow-up study of Alameda County residents." *American Journal of Epidemiology,* 1979, 109(2):186–204.
41. Berkman, L. F. "The role of social relations in health promotion." *Psychosomatic Medicine,* 1995, 57:245–54.
42. Berkman, L., and L. Breslow. *Health and Ways of Living: The Alameda County Study.* New York: Oxford University Press, 1983.
43. Reynolds, P., and G. A. Kaplan. "Social connections and risk for cancer: prospective evidence from the Alameda County Study." *Behavioral Medicine,* 1990, 16(3):101–10.
44. Reynolds, P., P. T. Boyd, and R. S. Blacklow. "The relationship between social ties and survival among black and white breast cancer patients. National Cancer Institute Black/White Cancer Survival Study Group." *Cancer Epidemiology, Biomarkers & Prevention,* 1994, 3(3):253–59.
45. Marshall, J. R., and D. P. Funch. "Social environment and breast cancer. A

cohort analysis of patient survival." *Cancer*, 1983, 52(8):1546–50.

46. House, J. S., C. Robbins, and H. L. Metzner. "The association of social relationships and activities with mortality: prospective evidence from the Tecumseh Community Health Study." *American Journal of Epidemiology*, 1982, 116(1):123–40.

47. Orth-Gomér, K., and J. V. Johnson. "Social network interaction and mortality. A six year follow-up study of a random sample of the Swedish population." *Journal of Chronic Diseases*, 1987, 40(10):949–57.

48. Hanson, B. S., S. O. Isacsson, L. Janzon, and S. E. Lindell. "Social network and social support influence mortality in elderly men. The prospective population study of 'Men born in 1914.' " *American Journal of Epidemiology*, 1989, 130(1):100–111.

49. Ruberman, W., E. Weinblatt, J. D. Goldberg, and B. S. Chaudhary. "Psychosocial influences on mortality after myocardial infarction." *New England Journal of Medicine*, 1984, 311(9): 552–59.

50. Kaplan, G. A., J. T. Salonen, R. D. Cohen, et al. "Social connections and

mortality from all causes and from cardiovascular disease: prospective evidence from eastern Finland." *American Journal of Epidemiology*, 1988, 128(2): 370–80.

51. Schoenbach, V. J., B. H. Kaplan, L. Fredman, and D. G. Kleinbaum. "Social ties and mortality in Evans County, Georgia." *American Journal of Epidemiology*, 1986, 123(4):577–91.

52. Kaplan, G. A. "Social contacts and ischaemic heart disease." *Annals of Clinical Research*, 1988, 20(1–2):131–36.

53. Seeman, T. E., L. F. Berkman, F. Kohout, et al. "Intercommunity variations in the association between social ties and mortality in the elderly. A comparative analysis of three communities." *Annals of Epidemiology*, 1993, 3(4):325–35.

54. Ortmeyer, C. F. "Variations in mortality, morbidity, and health care by marital status." In L. L. Erhardt and J. E. Beln, eds., *Mortality and Morbidity in the United States*. Cambridge: Harvard University Press, 1974, pp. 159–84.

55. Ernster, V. L., S. T. Sacks, S. Selvin, et al. "Cancer incidence by marital status." *Journal of the National Cancer Institute*, 1979, 63:567–85.

56. Goodwin, J. S., W. C. Hunt, C. R. Key, and J. M. Samet. "The effect of marital status on stage, treatment, and survival of cancer patients." *Journal of the American Medical Association*, 1987, 3125–30.

57. Williams, R. B., J. C. Barefoot, R. M. Califf, et al. "Prognostic importance of social and economic resources among medically treated patients with angiographically documented coronary artery disease." *Journal of the American Medical Association*, 1992, 267(4):520–24.

58. Chandra, V., M. Szklo, R. Goldberg, et al. "The impact of marital status on survival after an acute myocardial infarction: a population-based study." *American Journal of Epidemiology*, 1983, 117(3):320–25.

59. Wiklund, I., A. Oden, H. Sanne, et al. "Prognostic importance of somatic and psychosocial variables after a first myocardial infarction." *American Journal of Epidemiology*, 1988, 128(4):786–95.

60. Blazer, D. G. "Social support and mortality in an elderly community population." *American Journal of Epidemiology*, 1982, 115(5):684–94.

61. Case, R. B., A. J. Moss, N. Case, et al. "Living alone after myocardial in-

farction. Impact on prognosis." *Journal of the American Medical Association*, 1992, 267(4):515–19.

62. Penninx, B. W., T. van Tilburg, D. M. Kriegsman, et al. "Effects of social support and personal coping resources on mortality in older age: the Longitudinal Aging Study Amsterdam." *American Journal of Epidemiology*, 1997, 146(6): 510–19.

63. Woloshin, S., et al. *Journal of General Internal Medicine*, 1997, 12:613–18.

64. Berkman, L. F., L. Leo-Summers, and R. I. Horwitz. "Emotional support and survival after myocardial infarction. A prospective, population-based study of the elderly." *Annals of Internal Medicine*, 1992, 117(12):1003–9.

65. Marmot, M. G., S. L. Syme, A. Kagan, et al. "Epidemiologic studies of coronary heart disease and stroke in Japanese men living in Japan, Hawaii and California: prevalence of coronary and hypertensive heart disease and associated risk factors." *American Journal of Epidemiology*, 1975, 102(6):514–25.

66. Marmot, M. G., and S. L. Syme. "Acculturation and coronary heart disease in Japanese-Americans." *American Journal of Epidemiology*, 1976, 104(3):

225–47.

67. Oxman, T. E., D. H. Freeman, Jr., and E. D. Manheimer. "Lack of social participation or religious strength and comfort as risk factors for death after cardiac surgery in the elderly." *Psychosomatic Medicine*, 1995, 57:5–15.

68. Spiegel, D., J. R. Bloom, H. C. Kraemer, E. Gottheil. "Effect of psychosocial treatment on survival of patients with metastatic breast cancer." *The Lancet*, 1989, ii: 888–91.

69. Siegel, B. *Love, Medicine, & Miracles*. New York: Harper and Row, 1986.

70. Spiegel, D. *Living Beyond Limits: New Hope and Help for Facing Life-Threatening Illness*. New York: Times Books, 1993.

71. Fawzy, F. I., N. W. Fawzy, C. S. Hyun, et al. "Malignant melanoma: Effects of an early structured psychiatric intervention, coping, and affective state on recurrence and survival six years later." *Archives of General Psychiatry*, 1993, 50:681–89.

72. Cunningham, A. J., and C. V. I. Edmonds. "Group psychological therapy for cancer patients: a point of view, and discussion of the hierarchy of options." *International Journal of Psychiatry in*

Medicine, 1996, 26:51–82.

73. Shekelle, R. B., W. J. Raynor, and A. M. Ostfeld. "Personality and risk of cancer: 20-year follow-up of the Western Electric Study." *Psychosomatic Medicine*, 1981, 43:117–25.

74. Shekelle, R. B., W. J. Raynor, Jr., A. M. Ostfeld, et al. "Psychological depression and 17-year risk of death from cancer." *Psychosomatic Medicine*, 1981, 43(2):117–25.

75. Funch, D. P., and J. Marshall. "The role of stress, social support and age in survival from breast cancer." *Journal of Psychosomatic Research*, 1983, 27(1): 77–83.

76. Miller, T. Q., T. W. Smith, C. W. Turner, et al. "A meta-analytic review of research on hostility and physical health." *Psychological Bulletin*, 1996, 119:322–48.

77. Review Panel on Coronary-Prone Behavior and Coronary Heart Disease. "Coronary-prone behavior and coronary heart disease: a critical review." *Circulation*, 1978, 65:1199–1215.

78. Ornish, D. *Dr. Dean Ornish's Program for Reversing Heart Disease*. New York: Random House, 1990; Ballantine Books, 1992.

79. Frasure-Smith, N., and R. Prince. "Long-term follow-up of the Ischemic Heart Disease Life Stress Monitoring Program." *Psychosomatic Medicine,* 1989, 51(5):485–513.
80. Olsen, O. "Impact of social networks on cardiovascular mortality in middle-aged Danish men." *Journal of Epidemiology and Community Health,* 1993, 47:176–80.
81. Kaplan, G. A., J. T. Salonen, R. D. Cohen, et al. "Social connections and mortality from all causes and from cardiovascular disease: prospective evidence from eastern Finland." *American Journal of Epidemiology,* 1988, 128(2): 370–80.
82. Friedman, M., C. E. Thoresen, J. J. Gill, et al. "Alteration of type A behavior and its effect on cardiac recurrences in post myocardial infarction patients: summary results of the recurrent coronary prevention project." *American Heart Journal,* 1986, 112(4):653–65.
83. Powell, L., and C. Thoresen. "Modifying the type A behavior pattern." In J. Blumenthal and D. McKee, eds. *Applications in Behavioral Medicine and Health Psychology: A Clinician's Source Book.* Sarasota: Professional Resources

Exchange, 1987, p. 202.

84. Green, J., and R. Shellenberger. "The healing energy of love." *Alternative Therapies in Health and Medicine*, 1996, 2:46–56.

85. Friedman, M., and D. Ulmer. *Treating Type A Behavior*. New York: Random House, 1984, pp. 128–29.

86. Barefoot, J. C., I. C. Siegler, J. B. Nowlin, et al. "Suspiciousness, health, and mortality: a follow-up study of 500 older adults." *Psychosomatic Medicine*, 1987, 49(5):450–57.

87. Cohen, S., W. J. Doyle, D. P. Skoner, et al. "Social ties and susceptibility to the common cold." *Journal of the American Medical Association*, 1997, 277:1940–44.

88. Kiecolt-Glaser, J., et al. The Fourth International Congress of Behavioral Medicine, Washington, D.C., 1996.

89. Kiecolt-Glaser, J., et al. *Psychosomatic Medicine*, 1993, 55(5):395–409.

90. McClelland, D. C., and C. Kirshnit. "The effect of motivational arousal through films on salivary immuno-globulin A." *Psychology and Health*, 1988, 2:31–52.

91. McClelland, D. C. "Motivational factors in health and disease." *American*

Psychologist, 1989, 44(4):675–83.

92. Dreher, H. *The Immune Power Personality*. New York: Dutton Books, 1995.

93. Hoffman, S., and M. C. Hatch. "Stress, social support and pregnancy outcome: a reassessment based on recent research." *Paediatric & Perinatal Epidemiology*, 1996, 10(4):380–405.

94. Nuckolls, K. B., J. C. Cassel, and B. H. Kaplan. "Psychosocial assets, life crisis, and prognosis of pregnancy." *American Journal of Epidemiology*, 1972, 95:431–41.

95. Boyce, W. T., C. Schaefer, and C. Uitti. "Permanence and change: psychosocial factors in the outcome of adolescent pregnancy." *Social Science & Medicine*, 1985, 21(11):1279–87.

96. Boyce, W. T. "Stress and child health: an overview." *Pediatric Annals*, 1985, 14(8):539–42.

97. Sosa, R., J. Kennel, and M. Klaus. "The effect of a supportive companion on perinatal problems, length of labor and mother-infant interactions." *New England Journal of Medicine*, 1980, 305:597–600.

98. Berkman, L. F. "The relationship of social networks and social support to morbidity and mortality." In S. Cohen,

S. L. Syme, eds., *Social Support and Health*. Orlando: Academic Press, 1985.

99. Kennell, J., M. Klaus, S. McGrath, et al. "Continuous emotional support during labor in a US hospital. A randomized controlled trial." *Journal of the American Medical Association*, 1991, 265(17):2197–201.

100. Collins, N. L., C. Dunkel-Schetter, M. Lobel, et al. "Social support in pregnancy: Psychosocial correlates of birth outcomes and postpartum depression." *Journal of Personality and Social Psychology*, 1993, 65:1243–58.

101. Reeb, K. A., A. V. Graham, S. J. Zyzanski, and G. C. Kitson. "Predicting low birthweight and complicated labor in urban black women: a biopsychosocial perspective." *Social Science in Medicine*, 1987, 25:1321–27.

102. Molfese, V. J., M. C. Bricker, L. Manion, et al. "Stress in pregnancy: the influence of psychological and social mediators in perinatal experiences." *Journal of Psychosomatic Obstetrics and Gynecology*, 1987, 6:33–42.

103. Mutale, T., F. Creed, M. Maresh, and L. Hunt. "Live events and low birthweight." *British Journal of Obstetrics and*

Gynecology, 1991, 98:166–72.

104. Peacock, J. L., J. M. Bland, and H. R. Anderson. "Preterm delivery: effects of socioeconomic factors, psychological stress, smoking, alcohol, and caffeine." *British Medical Journal*, 1995, 311: 531–36.

105. Norbeck, J. S., and N. J. Anderson. "Psychosocial predictors of pregnancy outcomes in low-income black, Hispanic, and white women." *Nursing Research*, 1989, 38:204–9.

106. Friedmann, E., and S. A. Thomas. "Pet ownership, social support, and one-year survival after acute myocardial infarction in the Cardiac Arrhythmia Suppression Trial (CAST)." *American Journal of Cardiology*, 1995, 76:1213–17.

107. Friedmann, E., A. H. Katcher, J. J. Lynch, et al. "Animal companions and one-year survival of patients after discharge from a coronary care unit." *Public Health Reports*, 1980, 95:307–12.

108. Siegel, J. M. "Stressful life events and use of physician services among the elderly: the moderating role of pet ownership." *Journal of Personality and Social Psychology*, 1990, 58:1081–86.

109. Friedmann, E., A. H. Katcher, S. A.

Thomas, et al. "Social interaction and blood pressure: Influence of animal companions." *Journal of Nervous and Mental Disease*, 1983, 171:461–65.

110. Allen, K. M., J. T. Blascovich, and R. M. Kelsey. "Presence of human friends and pet dogs as moderators of autonomic responses to stress in women." *Journal of Personality and Social Psychology*, 1991, 61:582–89.

111. Nerem, R. M., M. J. Levesque, J. F. Cornhill. "Social environment as a factor in diet-induced atherosclerosis." *Science*, 1980, 208(4451):1475–76.

112. Skinner, J. E., J. T. Lie, and M. L. Entman. "Modification of ventricular fibrillation latency following coronary."

113. Lynch, J. J., S. A. Thomas, D. A. Paskewitz, et al. "Human contact and cardiac arrhythmia in a coronary care unit." *Psychosomatic Medicine*, 1977, 39(3):188–92.

114. Lynch, J. J. *The Broken Heart: The Medical Consequences of Loneliness*. New York: Basic Books, 1977.

115. Justice, B. *Who Gets Sick*. Los Angeles: Tarcher Books, 1988.

116. Pilisuk, M., and S. H. Parks. *The Healing Web*. Hanover, NH: University

Press of New England, 1986.
117. Shumaker, S. A., and S. M. Czajkowski, eds. *Social Support and Cardiovascular Disease*. New York: Plenum Press, 1994.
118. Hafen, B. Q., K. J. Karren, K. J. Frandsen, and N. L. Smith. *Mind/Body Health*. Needham Heights, MA: Allyn & Bacon, 1996.
119. Totman, R. *Social Causes of Illness*. New York: Pantheon Books, 1979.
120. Cohen, S., and S. L. Syme, eds. *Social Support and Health*. Orlando: Academic Press, 1985.

Chapter 4: Pathways to Love and Intimacy

1. Billings, J., L. Scherwitz, R. Sullivan, and D. Ornish. "Group support therapy in the Lifestyle Heart Trial." In S. Scheidt and R. Allan, eds., *Heart and Mind: The Emergence of Cardiac Psychology*. Washington, D.C.: American Psychological Association, 1996, pp. 233–53.
2. Berry, D. S., and J. W. Pennebaker. "Nonverbal and verbal emotional expression and health." *Psychother. Psychosom.*, 1993, 59:11–19.

3. Pennebaker, J. W., and J. R. Susman. "Disclosure of traumas and psychosomatic processes." *Soc. Sci. Med.*, 1988, 26:327–32.

4. Petrie, K. J., R. J. Booth, J. W. Pennebaker, et al. "Disclosure of trauma and immune response to a hepatitis B vaccination program." *Journal of Consulting and Clinical Psychology*, 1995, 63:787–92.

5. Pennebaker, J. W., C. F. Hughes, R. C. O'Heeron. "The psychophysiology of confession." *Journal of Personality and Social Psychology*, 1987, 52: 781–93.

6. Pennebaker, J. W., S. D. Barger, and J. Tiebout. "Disclosure of traumas and health among Holocaust survivors." *Psychosomatic Medicine*, 1989, 51: 577–89.

7. Francis, M. E., and J. W. Pennebaker. "Putting stress into words." *American Journal of Health Promotion*, 1992, 6:280–87.

8. Pennebaker, J. W. *Opening Up: The Healing Power of Confiding in Others.* New York: William Morrow, 1990, pp. 118–19.

9. *Gates of Repentance.* New York: Central Conference of American Rabbis,

1978, p. 335.

10. Luke 23:34.

11. House, J. S., K. R. Landis, and D. Umberson. "Social relationships and health." *Science*, 1988, 241:540–45.

12. Moen, P., D. Dempster-McClain, and R. M. Williams. "Successful aging." *American Journal of Sociology*, 1993, 97:1612–38.

13. McClelland, D. C., and C. Kirshnit. "The effect of motivational arousal through films on salivary immuno-globulin A." *Psychology and Health*, 1988, 2:31–52.

14. Lynch, J. J. *The Broken Heart: The Medical Consequences of Loneliness.* New York: Basic Books, 1977; Baltimore: Bancroft Press, 1998.

15. Exodus 3:13

16. Satchidananda, S. *The Yoga Sutras of Patanjali.* Buckingham, VA: Integral Yoga Publications, 1990.

17. Luke 17:21

18. Mitchell, S., ed. *The Enlightened Mind.* New York: HarperCollins Publishers, 1991.

19. Ibid.

20. Ibid.

21. Huxley, A. *The Perennial Philosophy.* New York: Harper & Row, 1945.

22. Leviticus 19:18
23. Yeats, W. B., and S. P. Swami. *The Ten Principal Upanishads*. New York: Macmillan, 1937. Also found in S. Mitchell, ed., *The Enlightened Mind*.
24. Shantideva. *The Way of the Bodhisattva*. Boston: Shambhala Publishers, 1997.
25. Ibid., chapter 8, verse 129.
26. Mitchell, S. *The Gospel According to Jesus*. New York: HarperCollins Publishers, 1991.
27. Colt, G. H. "The Magic of Touch." *Life* magazine, August 1997, p. 55.
28. Montagu, A. *Touching: The Human Significance of the Skin*. New York: Harper & Row, 1986.
29. Field, T. "Massage therapy for infants and children." *Journal of Developmental & Behavioral Pediatrics*, 1995, 16(2): 105–11.
30. Ironson, G., T. Field, F. Scafidi, et al. "Massage therapy is associated with enhancement of the immune system's cytotoxic capacity." *International Journal of Neuroscience*, 1996, 84(1–4):205–17.
31. Jourard, S. M. "An exploratory study of body-accessibility." *British Journal of Social & Clinical Psychology*, 1966, 5(3):221–31.
32. Quinn, J. "Therapeutic touch and a

healing way." *Alternative Therapies in Health and Medicine,* 1996, 2(4):69–75.

33. Quinn, J. F., and A. J. Strelkauskas. "Psychoimmunologic effects of therapeutic touch on practitioners and recently bereaved recipients: a pilot study." *Advances in Nursing Science,* 1993, 15(4):13–26.

34. Kornfield, J. *A Path with Heart.* New York: Bantam Books, 1993.

35. Ibid.

Selected Bibliography

Anand, Margo. *The Art of Sexual Ecstasy.* New York: Tarcher/Putnam Books, 1989.

Borysenko, Joan. *A Woman's Book of Life.* New York: Riverhead Books, 1996.

Carter, Rosalynn. *Helping Yourself Help Others.* New York: Times Books, 1994.

Cohen, Sheldon, and S. Leonard Syme. *Social Support and Health.* Orlando, Florida: Academic Press, 1985.

Coles, Robert. *The Call of Stories: Teaching and the Moral Imagination.* Boston: Houghton Mifflin, 1989.

Cortis, Bruno. *Heart and Soul.* New York: Villard Books, 1995.

Dass, Ram, and Marabai Bush. *Compassion in Action.* New York: Bell Tower, 1992.

Dossey, Larry. *Healing Words.* New York: HarperCollins Publishers, 1993.

_____. *Meaning and Medicine.* New York: Bantam Books, 1991.

_____. *Prayer Is Good Medicine.* New York: HarperCollins Publishers, 1996.

Dreher, Henry. *The Immune Power Personality.* New York: The Penguin Group, 1995.

495

Fuller, Millard. *The Theology of the Hammer.* Macon, Georgia: Smyth & Helwys Publishing, Inc., 1994.

Goleman, Daniel. *Emotional Intelligence.* New York: Bantam Books, 1995.

Gray, John. *Men Are from Mars, Women Are from Venus.* New York: HarperCollins Publishers, 1992.

Hafen, Brent Q., Keith J. Karren, Kathryn J. Frandsen, and N. Lee Smith. *Mind/Body Health.* Needham Heights, Massachusetts: Allyn & Bacon, 1996.

Hanh, Thich Nhat. *The Miracle of Mindfulness.* Boston: Beacon Press, 1975.

His Holiness the Dalai Lama. *Healing Anger: The Power of Patience from a Buddhist Perspective.* Ithaca, New York: Snow Lion Publications, 1997.

_____. *The Power of Compassion.* London: Thorsons, 1995.

_____. *The Way to Freedom.* New York: HarperCollins Publishers, 1994.

Joy, Brugh. *Joy's Way.* New York: Putnam Books, 1979.

Justice, Blair. *Who Gets Sick.* Houston: Peak Press, 1987.

Kabat-Zinn, Jon. *Full Catastrophe Living.* New York: Delacorte Press, 1990.

_____. *Wherever You Go There You Are.* New York: Hyperion, 1994.

Keen, Sam. *To Love and Be Loved.* New York: Bantam Books, 1997.

Kesten, Deborah. *Feeding the Body, Nourishing the Soul.* Berkeley: Conari Press, 1997.

Kornfield, Jack. *Living Dharma: Teachings of Twelve Buddhist Masters.* Boston: Shambhala Publications, 1996.

_____. *A Path with Heart.* New York: Bantam Books, 1993.

Lasher, Margot. *The Art and Practice of Compassion.* New York: Tarcher/Putnam Books, 1992.

Levine, Stephen, and Ondrea Levine. *Embracing the Beloved.* New York: Doubleday, 1995.

Lynch, James J. *The Broken Heart.* New York: Basic Books, 1977; Baltimore: Bancroft Press, 1998.

_____. *The Language of the Heart.* New York: Basic Books, 1985; Baltimore: Bancroft Press, 1998.

Miller, Alice. *For Your Own Good.* New York: Noonday Publishing, 1983.

Miller, Ronald S. *As Above, So Below.* Los Angeles: Jeremy P. Tarcher, 1992.

Mitchell, Stephen. *The Enlightened Heart.* New York: HarperCollins Publishers, 1989.

_____. *The Enlightened Mind.* New York:

HarperCollins Publishers, 1991.

_____. *Parables and Portraits*. New York: HarperCollins Publishers, 1990.

Moss, Richard. *The I That Is We*. Berkeley: Celestial Arts, 1981.

Moyers, Bill. *Healing and the Mind*. New York: Doubleday, 1993.

Ornish, Dean. *Dr. Dean Ornish's Program for Reversing Heart Disease*. New York: Random House, 1990; Ballantine Books, 1991.

_____. *Eat More, Weigh Less*. New York: HarperCollins Publishers, 1993.

_____. *Everyday Cooking with Dr. Dean Ornish*. New York: HarperCollins Publishers, 1996.

_____. *Stress, Diet, & Your Heart*. New York: Holt, Rinehart and Winston, 1982; New American Library (Signet Books), 1983.

Ornstein, Robert, and David Sobel. *Healthy Pleasures*. New York: Addison-Wesley, 1989.

Pennebaker, James W. *Opening Up: The Healing Power of Confiding in Others*. New York: William Morrow & Co., Inc., 1990.

Pert, Candace. *Molecules of Emotion: Why We Feel the Way We Feel*. New York: Scribner Books/Simon & Schuster, 1997.

Pilisuk, Marc, and Susan Hillier Parks. *The Healing Web*. Hanover, New Hampshire: University Press of New England, 1986.

Remen, Rachel Naomi. *Kitchen Table Wisdom*. New York: Riverhead Books, 1996.

Rinpoche, Sogyal. *The Tibetan Book of Living and Dying*. New York: HarperCollins Publishers, 1992.

Satchidananda, Sri Swami. *The Golden Present*. Buckingham, Virginia: Integral Yoga Publications, 1987.

_____. *Pathway to Peace*. Buckingham, Virginia: Integral Yoga Publications, 1988.

_____. *Peace Is Within Our Reach*. Buckingham, Virginia: Integral Yoga Publications, 1985.

_____. *The Yoga Sutras of Patanjali*. Buckingham, Virginia: Integral Yoga Publications, 1990.

Scarf, Maggie. *Intimate Partners*. New York: Ballantine Books, 1987.

Shaffer, Carolyn, and Kristin Anundsen. *Creating Community Anywhere*. New York: Tarcher/Putnam Books, 1993.

Shantideva. *The Way of the Bodhisattva*. Boston: Shambhala Publications, Inc., 1997.

Shumaker, Sall A., and Susan M. Czajkowski. *Social Support and Cardiovascular*

Disease. New York: Plenum Press, 1994.

Sinatra, Stephen T. *Heartbreak & Heart Disease.* New Canaan: Keats Publishing, 1996.

Spiegel, David. *Living Beyond Limits.* New York: Ballantine Books, 1993.

Steindl-Rast, Brother David. *Gratefulness, the Heart of Prayer.* Ramsey, New Jersey: Paulist Press, 1984.

Tannen, Deborah. *You Just Don't Understand.* New York: Ballantine Books, 1990.

Thurman, Robert A. F. *Essential Tibetan Buddhism.* New York: HarperSanFrancisco, 1995.

Totman, Richard. *Social Causes of Illness.* New York: Pantheon Books, 1979.

Vivekananda. *Living at the Source.* Boston: Shambhala Publications, Inc., 1993.

Weil, Andrew. *Spontaneous Healing.* New York: Knopf, 1995.

Welwood, John. *Journey of the Heart.* New York: HarperCollins Publishers, 1990.

Williams, Virginia, and Redford Williams. *Lifeskills.* New York: Times Books, 1997.

Zaleski, Philip, and Paul Kaufman. *Gifts of the Spirit.* New York: HarperCollins Publishers, 1997.

About the Author

Dean Ornish, M.D., holds the Bucksbaum Chair in Preventive Medicine at the nonprofit Preventive Medicine Research Institute in Sausalito, California, which he founded in 1984. He is Clinical Professor of Medicine at the School of Medicine at the University of California, San Francisco, and a founder of the Center of Integrative Medicine there. He is also an attending physician at California Pacific Medical Center. Dr. Ornish received an M.D. from Baylor College of Medicine in Houston, was a clinical fellow in medicine at Harvard Medical School, and completed his internship and residency in internal medicine at the Massachusetts General Hospital in Boston.

For the past twenty years, Dr. Ornish has directed clinical research demonstrating — for the first time — that comprehensive lifestyle changes may begin to reverse even severe coronary heart disease, without drugs or surgery. He is the author of four bestselling books.

His research has been published in the *Journal of the American Medical Association*, the *Lancet, Circulation,* the *American Journal of Cardiology,* and elsewhere. A one-hour documentary of his work was broadcast on *NOVA,* the PBS science series, and was featured on Bill Moyers's PBS special *Healing and the Mind.* His work has been featured in virtually all major media.

Dr. Ornish has received several awards, including the 1996 Beckmann Medal from the German Society for Prevention and Rehabilitation of Cardiovascular Diseases, the U.S. Army Surgeon General Medal, and the 1994 outstanding young alumnus award from the University of Texas, Austin. He was recognized as one of the most interesting people of 1995 by *People* magazine and as one of the fifty most influential members of his generation by *Life* magazine.